TAPING TECHNIQUE

Theory and Practice

TAPING TECHNIQUE

Theory and Practice

Dr. C.S. Ram

Director—Physiotherapy
Institute of Technology and Science
Muradnagar
Ghaziabad - 201206 (UP)

PEEPEE

PUBLISHERS AND DISTRIBUTORS (P) LTD.

Taping Technique: Theory and Practice

Published by
Pawaninder P. Vij

Peepee Publishers and Distributors (P) Ltd.
Head Office: 160, Shakti Vihar, Pitam Pura
Delhi-110034 (India)

Correspondence Address: 7/31, First Floor, Ansari Road, Daryaganj
Post Box-7243, New Delhi-110002 (India)

Ph: 65195868, 23246245, 9811156083

e-mail: peepee160@yahoo.co.in

e-mail: peepee160@rediffmail.com

e-mail: peepee160@gmail.com

www.peepeepub.com

First Edition: **2011**

ISBN: 81-8445-066-4

Printed at
Lordson, C-5/19, Rana Pratap Bagh, Delhi-110 007

PREFACE

Taping Techniques by Dr. C.S. Ram is a treatise on practical application of adhesive taping.

The book provides exhaustive and elaborative explanation of the method of applying adhesive tapes for different injuries. Various joints of the human body which sustain injury have been dealt with. The book is a treasure trove of pictures on taping.

It is useful resource manual for physiotherapists practising especially in sports or orthopaedics field, coaches, sports medicine specialists, orthopaedic surgeons etc.

Dr. C.S. Ram

ACKNOWLEDGEMENTS

The development of this book is a dream come true for many persons. What started as a project culminated in the form of this book. It is the hard work of my team from I.T.S. College of Physiotherapy that has given shape to this book.

First and foremost I would like to thank Dr. Shristee Khushwah and Dr. Supriya Sharma, my students in M.P.T. program for the valuable contribution.

I would like to thank Dr. Gaurav Shori for the help rendered in guiding the project.

Special thanks are due to Dr. Mehtab Nayyar for proof reading the entire material despite her busy schedule.

Last but not the least I would like to thank the publishers Mr. Pawaninder P Vij and Mr. Anupam Vij for their patience in waiting for the project to complete. I would also like to thank the office staff of Peepee Publishers for presenting the book in the present form.

Dr. C.S. Ram

CONTRIBUTORS

Dr. Gaurav Shori
Asst. Prof.
I.T.S. College of Physiotherapy
Muradnagar
Ghaziabad - 201206 (UP)

Dr. Shrishtee Khushwah
Fitness Trainer
I.T.S. College of Physiotherapy
Muradnagar
Ghaziabad - 201206 (UP)

CONTENTS

1 INTRODUCTION AND HISTORY

Taping is described as the application of adhesive tape–elastic (stretch) or non-elastic (rigid) in order to provide support and protection to soft tissues and joints to minimize swelling and pain after injury.

If the tape is being applied by a physical therapist then a thorough examination of the problem would have to be undertaken. The application of tape is with the aim of limiting unwanted movement at a joint or offloading specific anatomical structures where a weakness has been identified. Because there are a huge number of structures that could require support there is no single definitive taping technique. Therefore, the taping featured in this book provides an outline for quick and effective taping methods, with a degree of improvement necessary for each specific problem.

2 Tools and Measures for Taping

ESSENTIAL TAPING TOOLS

1. Razor and soap.
2. Skin toughener spray.
3. Lubricating ointment.
4. Pads.
5. Under-wrap.
6. Adhesive elastic tape 7.5 cm (3 inch).
7. Bandage scissors.
8. Padding: felt or foam.
9. Elastic bandage 7.5 cm (3 inch),15 cm (6 inch).

ADDITIONAL ITEMS FOR FIELD KIT

1. Antiseptic lotion.
2. Ice and towel.
3. Pen, pencil and papers.
4. Cotton gauge and strips.

OPTIONAL SUPPLIES

1. Surgical gloves.
2. Instant cold packs.
3. Antibiotic ointment.
4. Antifungal spray.
5. Blister protectors.
6. Cotton-tipped applicators.
7. Tongue depressors.
8. Quick drying adhesive spray.
9. Waterproof tape.
10. Adhesive remover.
11. Tape cutters.
12. Nail clippers.

1. **Adhesive elastic tape:** This tape offers elasticity and adhesion, maintaining localized compression over a contusion. Keeping maximal pressure on sprain.
2. **Antiseptic lotion; antibiotic ointment; antifungal spray:** Useful as a secondary precaution in treating minor abrasions, blisters, lacerations, Apply to cleaned wounds prior to taping.
3. **Skin toughener spray:** Fast drying aerosol sprays forming a microscopic adhesive layer protecting skin from contact with tape irritants.
4. **Adhesive spray:** Quick drying adhesive sprays applied directly to the skin to keep tape from slipping.
5. **Under-wrap, pro-wrap, pre-wrap:** Applied to the taping area between "anchors", this thin foam material reduces the area of direct skin contact, protects skin from traction burns and from tape irritation. The use of under-wrap can be very helpful when taping bony areas which are particularly susceptible to skin blisters and tape cuts.
6. **Lubricating ointment:** Viscous lubricating ointments used to decrease friction between tape and skin.
7. **Heel and lace pads:** Thin foam squares used in areas where there is a likelihood of friction under the taping–such as the laces of anterior ankle and the heel.
8. **Sterile gauze pads:** Pads with a non-stick surface are useful for open wounds as well as to cleanse abrasions and lacerations with antiseptic solution.

9. **Elastic bandages:** A variety of different widths needed (3 inch and 6 inch).

   6 inch: Support for thigh and groin strains, compression on soft tissue injuries.

   4 inch: Support for ankle sprains, devising a makeshift sling.

   3 inch: Small ankles, large wrists, distal joints.

   2 inch: Wrist sprains, children's injury.

10. **Padding foam:** It is a thin sheet made up of dense foam. It is useful when taping a bruised area: i.e. when taping a bruised tibia a layer of padding protects the injured area.
11. **Plastic adhesive stirrups:** Available in a variety of widths and lengths.
12. Tape cutters.
13. Bandage scissors.
14. **Pen or pencil paper** (notebook preferable).
15. **Surgical gloves:** Non sterile, disposable rubber gloves.

Taping is to provide protection and support for an injured part while permitting optimal functional movement. Taping enhances healing by allowing early activity within carefully controlled ranges. Taping also permits an earlier return to play or competition by protecting the area from further injury and avoiding compensatory injuries elsewhere.

3 TAPING OBJECTIVES

PURPOSES OF TAPING

- Support an injured structure.
- Limit harmful movements.
- Allow pain free functional movements.
- Permit early resumption of activities.

BENEFITS OF TAPING

- Increase of circulation through movement.
- Controlling oedema.
- Prevent:
  a. Worsening of initial injury.
  b. Compensatory injury to adjacent parts.
  c. Atrophy from non use.
- Allows:
  a. Continued body conditioning and strength gain during post-injury in activity.
  b. Maintenance of ability to react often lost due to inhibitive factors (pain, fear of re-injury).

TAPING can only be truly beneficial if the injury is properly assessed and the appropriate technique is utilized. An inappropriate tape job can place strain on associated areas and cause blisters or irritation, and in some cases, increases the severity of the injury and cause further damage to surrounding structures.

PRE-TAPING CONSIDERATIONS

By using the mnemonic **S.U.P.P.O.R.T.** to review the goals of effective taping, the taper can quickly run through a critical checklist before choosing the best technique and correlative materials for that particular injury.

SWELLING must be controlled by adequate padding and /or compression to prevent fluids from accumulating (oedema) and to ensure the best environment for tissue regeneration and repair.

UNDUE STRESS to the injured region must be prevented so as to reduce the possibility of additional injury or of increasing the severity of the injury.

PROTECTION of the area from further soft tissue damage (i.e. bruises, blisters and tape cuts) by using pads lubricants and other protective materials.

PAIN and discomfort must be minimized by supporting the injured part, by controlling unnecessary or excessive movement, and by taking care not to cause further irritation to the injured tissues.

OPTIMAL healing and tissue repair can be enhanced through correctly applying tape, keeping the range of motion within safe limits, and maintaining continuous compression.

REHABILITATION of the tissues to a fully functional state (joint mobility, soft tissue flexibility, muscle strength, ligament stability and proprioception) must be considered when choosing the taping technique adaptation for the appropriate stage of rehabilitation.

THERAPEUTIC CARE in the early stages of treatment is critical for a rapid recovery. Treatment may include the application of electrical modalities (ultrasound, laser, interferential electrotherapy, muscle stimulation, etc.) to control pain and swelling as well as to promote rapid healing.

POST-TAPING CONSIDERATION

In addition to being aware of the purposes of a particular taping application, there are conditions or situations to observe or to avoid after the taping is completed. The mnemonic **P.R.E.C.A.U.T.I.O.N.** will help recall several points important to post taping care.

PREMATURE participation in an activity which involves the injured part must be avoided. A major mistake many athletes makes is returning to action too soon. Such activity delays healing, an often results in reinjury to the weakened structure as well as damage to compensatory areas.

RANGE OF MOTION should be restricted but maintained as close as possible to the norm for the body part involved. Severe limitation of motion can result in an overextension of surrounding or compensatory structures. Permitting to free a range of motion will not adequately protect the tissue involved and will leave them prone to further injury.

EXPERT opinion must be obtained when any serious injury, particularly if a fracture or dislocation is suspected.

CIRCULATION in the injured area must be monitored for any sign of constrictions. Pressure bandage must be checked regularly.

ALLERGIES AND SKIN IRRITATIONS should be observed. The more serious degree of allergic reaction results in localized blistering, welts, pustules, rashes and pain. Simple irritation is generally a less severe reaction of reddened skin or small blisters.

UNDUE DEPENDENCY ON THE TAPING is a psychological danger which may arise when the athlete thinks he cannot perform without taping. In such cases the injured area may not return to its pre-injury performance level. Associated with this inaction, the athlete may have to spend unnecessary time in physiotherapy overcoming the results of excessive or prolonged taping.

TENDON, MUSCLE AND BODY PROMINENCES must be treated with special care and attention so as to avoid pressure built-up and friction.

ICE should not be applied to an injured part that is to be immediately subjected to taping. The temporary reduction of tissue volume due to icing will result in a taping that tightens progressively as the body parts warms up. Also, an athlete may have reduced skin sensation after icing, and tissue injury can result from such sensory loss.

ONLY top quality supplies should be used in order to ensure a consistently high standard of tape application.

NERVE conduction and local sensation may be interfered with by secondary inflammation or by the taping job itself. It is essential to evaluate the level of sensation prior to taping so that factors altering sensation can be assessed properly.

4 General Guidelines for Taping

GENERAL GUIDELINES FOR TAPING

Choosing the correct tape for a specific taping job: Choosing the right type of tape depends on the actual structure involved and whether the taping job involves padding, support, restraint or compression.

Elastic tape is used for contractile tissue injuries (i.e. muscles, tendons). Elastic tape is preferable in these instances because it gives stretch with support and a graduated resistance, yet limits full stretch of the muscle or tendon. Elastic tape should also be used for specific compression taping requiring localized pressure.

Non elastic tape is used to support injuries of non contractile structures (i.e. ligaments) non elastic tape reinforces the joint in the same way the ligaments would, thereby increasing joint stability.

TAPING APPLICATION

The person applying tape to an injury must modify the application to suit the circumstances specific to each situation. In taping procedures, protective layers with a lubricant should be used in areas particularly susceptible to irritation from taping, such as the back of heel, ankles, hamstring tendons and knee.

TAPING TECHNIQUES

The two main techniques used in applying tape are commonly referred as **strip taping** and smooth **roll.**

"Strip" taping employs one short strip of tape at a time, in very specific directions and with highly controlled tension.

"Smooth roll" refers to use of a single, continuous, uninterrupted winding of a piece of tape.

	Advantages	Disadvantages
Strips	Accurate tension tape applied only where needed	Requires time and practice.
Smooth roll	Quick to apply	Difficult to control tension.
	Useful when taping an entire team	Tendency to use too much tape.

QUALITY CONTROL: WHILE THE TAPING IS IN PROGRESS, MONITOR THESE POINTS

- Is effective compression being maintained without loss of circulation?
- Is the tape adhering properly?
- Is the injured structure being properly supported by the technique chosen?
- Are the supporting strips adequately tight?

Monitoring the results: Is the taping effective?

Follow these steps only when the tape job has been completed:

- Gently manually stress the joint movement to check for adequate limitation at the extremes of range of motion and in the direction of the injury.
- Check for stability of the joint and of the taping strips. The athlete should experience no pain during these tests.
- Further testing of the finished taping procedures involves functional tests in sport-specific movements as well as action and/or range of motion.

FUNCTIONAL TESTING: CAN THE ATHLETE SAFELY ENGAGE IN HIS SPORT?

Before the athlete can return to the playing field, it is necessary to thoroughly evaluate the taping relative to performance of sport-specific skills and movements. These tests, performed in order of increasing difficulty and stress to the joints, should be assessed by medical personnel.

TAPE REMOVAL

When a tape application is no longer required, removal of the tape job must be done carefully. The "tear – it – of – quick – before – you – know – it!" temptation should be avoided. This method causes skin damage jeopardizing subsequent or follow-up taping applications.

For speed and ease of tape removal, bandage scissors or special tape cutters should be used so as to avoid damage to skin and other sensitive structures in the area.

The preferred method is to first cut the tape: using the blunt tip of the scissors, ease the skin away from the adhering tape, forming a "tunnel" to facilitate cutting.

The tape is then peeled off slowly and gently, while pressing down on the exposed skin and pulling the tape back on itself, parallel–not perpendicular-to the surface of the skin.

USEFUL MNEMONIC

Before beginning any taping procedure it is important to properly assess the injured region in order to determine the most appropriate treatment and taping application.

The following material is presented in a format designed to facilitate a simple, quick method of assessment of injury in three areas: sprains, strains, contusion.

USING THE MNEMONIC T.E.S.T.S IN ASSESSING INJURED STRUCTURES

TERMINOLOGY

Proper names, synonyms and other pertinent information for identifying an injury or condition.

ETIOLOGY

Relative mechanisms, causative factors, prevalence.

SYMPTOMS

- Subjective complaints of the injured athlete including a description of the injury.
- Objective physical findings which can be measured by the taper.

TREATMENT

Includes early and later phases of first aid, physiotherapy, taping; medical follow-up when necessary.

SEQUELAE

Possible complications that can result if the original condition is left untreated, or is poorly treated, or if adequate expert medical follow-up is not pursued.

5 KEY TAPING TECHNIQUES

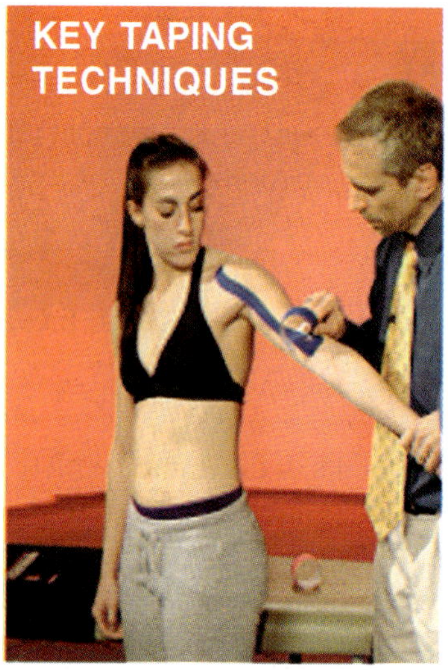

Most taping applications are variations on basic key taping strategies. The differences in taping technique lie in the manner and direction of tape and the type of taping material utilized. Each particular taping strategy has to meet the multiple requirements of a particular sport, the type of athlete has sustained.

The strips illustrated include:

- Anchors.
- Stirrups.
- Vertical.
- "Butterfly" or check–rein.
- Locks.
- Figure–8.
- Compression.
- Closing–up.

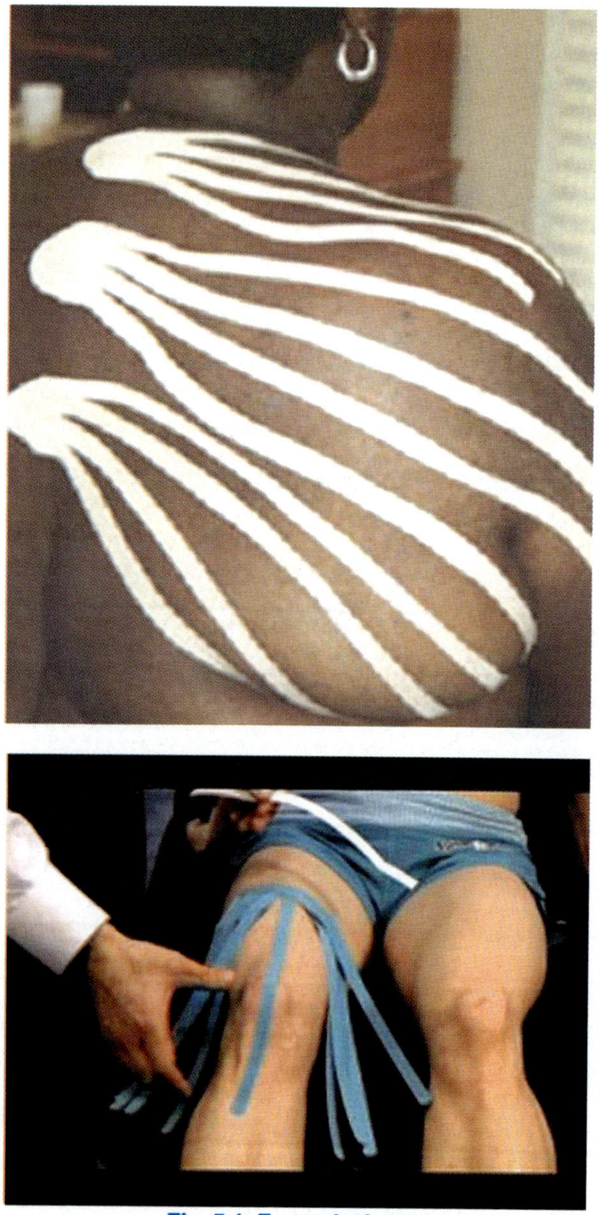

Fig. 5.1: Fanned stirrups

TAPE RIPPING (Figs. 5.2 and 5.3)

Tape ripping is an acquired skill and not as easy as it sounds. The steps shown in the two photographs will be useful in learning this practical skill.

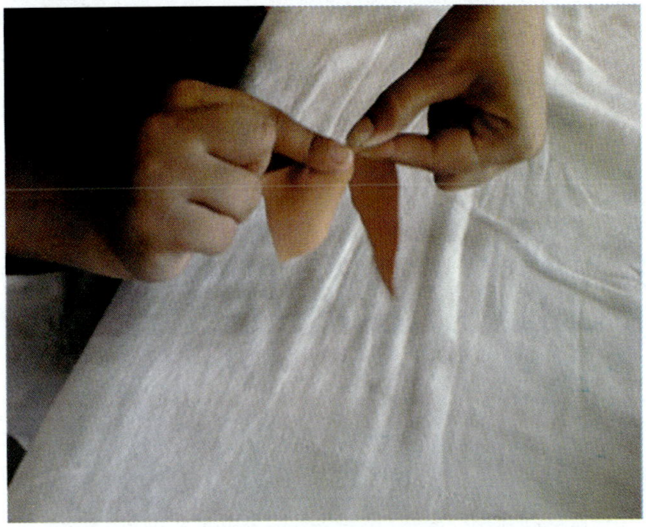

Fig. 5.2

1. Pinch the tape edge firmly with the thumb nails adjacent (back to back and perpendicular to the tape).

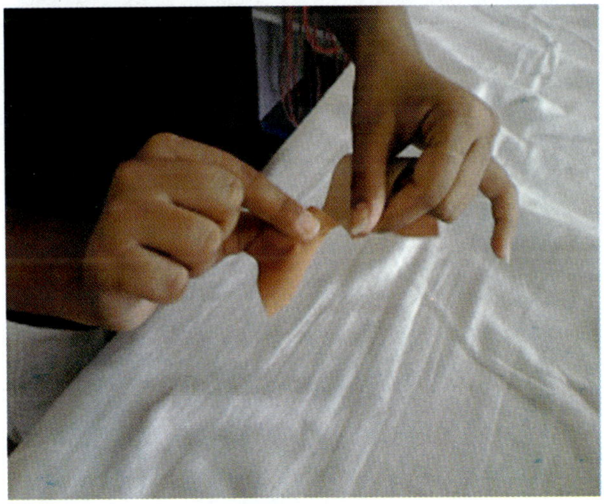

Fig. 5.3

2. Make a sudden jerking movements by sharply shearing your hands in opposite directions while maintaining tension on the tape edge.

PREPARATION OF PRACTICE STRIPS (Figs. 5.4 to 5.6)

To acquire taping skills, practice strips should be prepared. Because the precise application of Figure of 8 and locking strips are tricky to learn, it is advisable to apply numerous practice strips to perfect the technique.

This practice strip can be stuck to the limb as though it were a regular strip and the various complicated techniques can be practiced without wasting tape. With the "takeoff" angle and the degree on the lateral shearing, the taper can learn to accommodate for the varieties of ankle shapes and thickness. It is important to be able to control the direction of the strip and thus adapt the final supporting result.

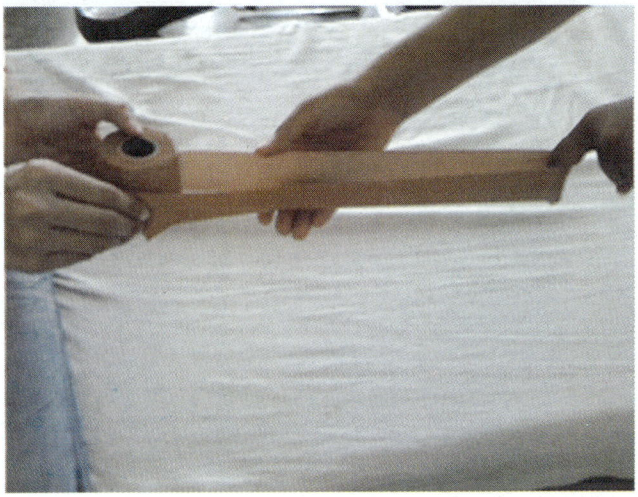

Fig. 5.4

1. Unroll 1 meter of tape and have a helper hold it at one end.
2. Hold the tape with two fingers (slightly separated) with your left hand while your helper unrolls another 1 meter of tape.

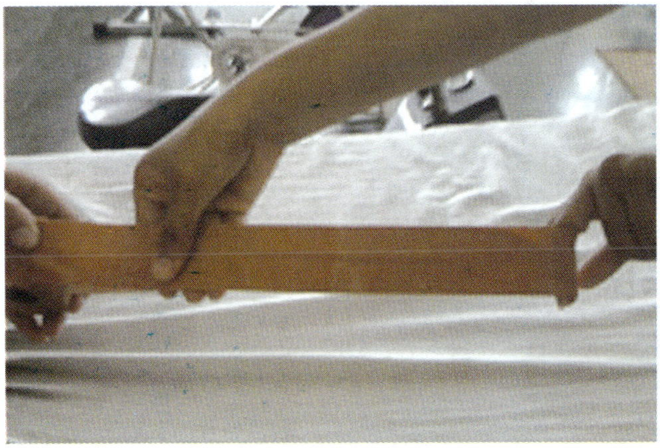

Fig. 5.5

3. Guide these two pieces of parallel tape (sticky side in) so that they meet without overlapping.
4. While maintaining tension on the tape gently presses one strip against the other throughout the length of the tape while controlling the tension to avoid wrinkles and overlapping.

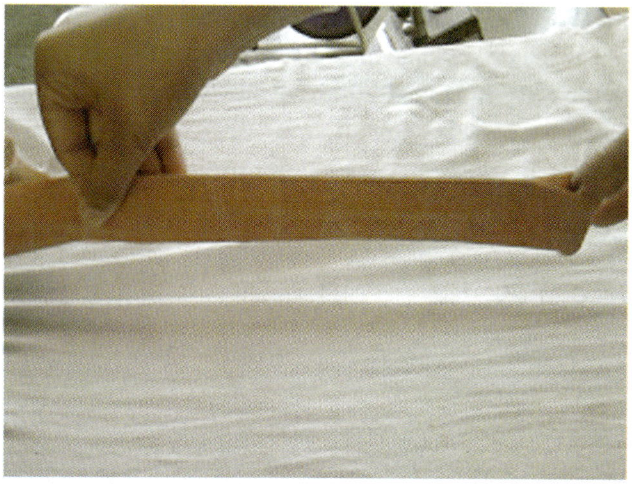

Fig. 5.6

5. Remove your fingers from the loop end of the tape and stick the sides together.
6. Finish sticking the other end of the tape and remove from the roll leaving one side 15 cm (6 ft) longer than the original piece with one sticky side.

COMMONLY USED TAPE STRIPS (Figs. 5.7(a) and (b))

Anchors description: The first tape strips applied for each tape job. They may be either nonelastic or elastic tape, depending on expansion requirements of the underlying structures.

Purpose: To form a stable base for subsequent supporting strips or tape.

Method: Place these tape strips around the circumference of the limb to be supported, both above and below the injury. They must be placed directly on the skin, and must follow anatomical contours for optimal adherence.

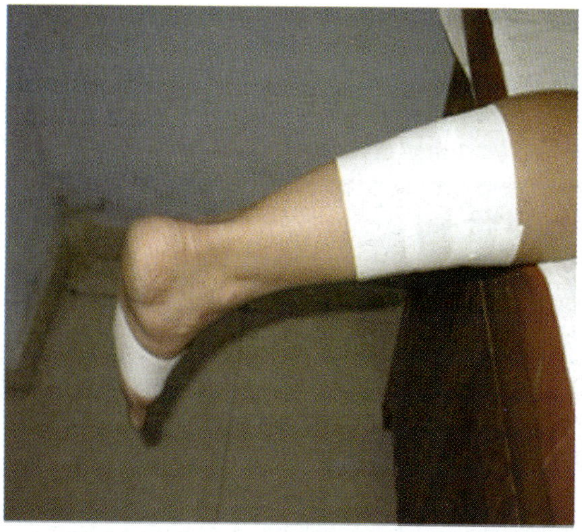

Fig. 5.7(a): Non-elastic tape anchors

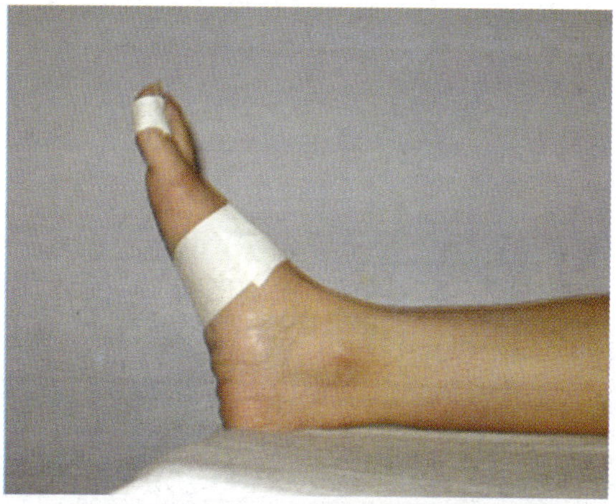

Fig. 5.7(b): Non-elastic tape anchors

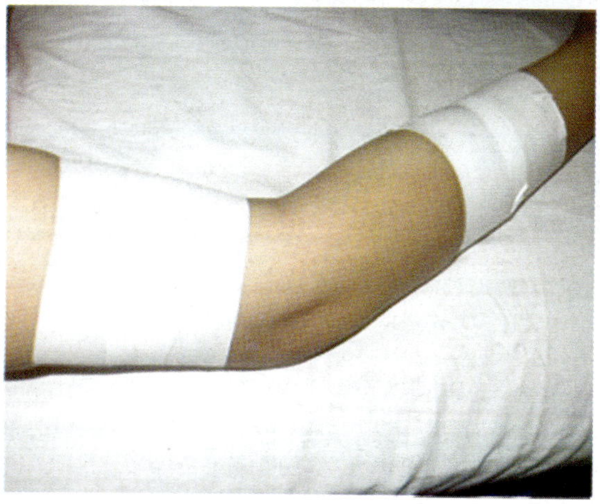

Fig. 5.8: Elastic tape anchors

STIRRUPS (Figs. 5.9(a) - (b))

Description: A U-shaped loop of non elastic tape.

Purpose: To directly support an injured ligament.

Method: Place the tape so that a lateral and a medial component give stability. Pull the tape tighter on the injured side.

> **NOTE**: Tension must be maintained until the strip is firmly attached.

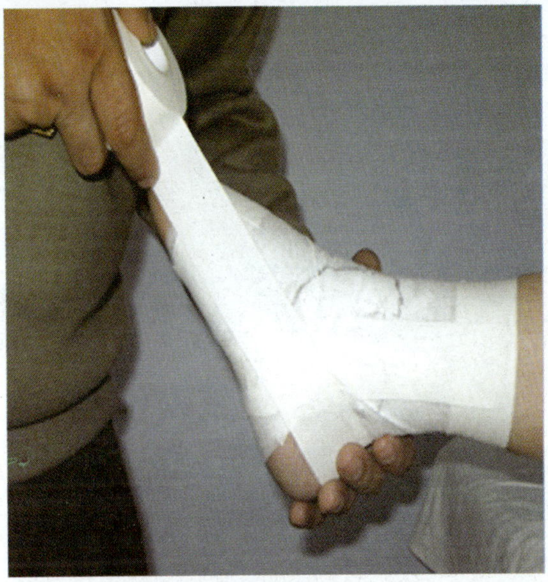

Fig. 5.9(a)

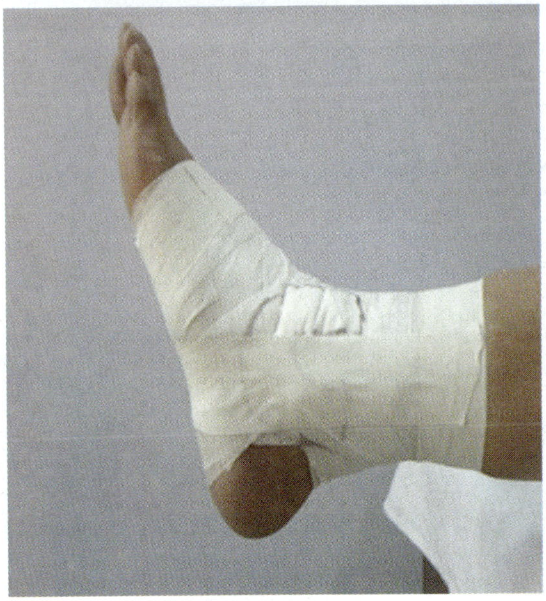

Fig. 5.9(b)

VERTICAL STRIPS (Figs. 5.10(a) - (b))

Description: Non-elastic tape strips applied under tension from one anchor to the other.

Purpose: To limit lateral mobility by drawing the distal segment of the injured structure towards the proximal.

Method: Affix one end of vertical strips to distal anchor and apply tension over the injured structure while affixing tape to the proximal anchor.

> **NOTE:** Proper poisoning of the injured limb is crucial to effective application.

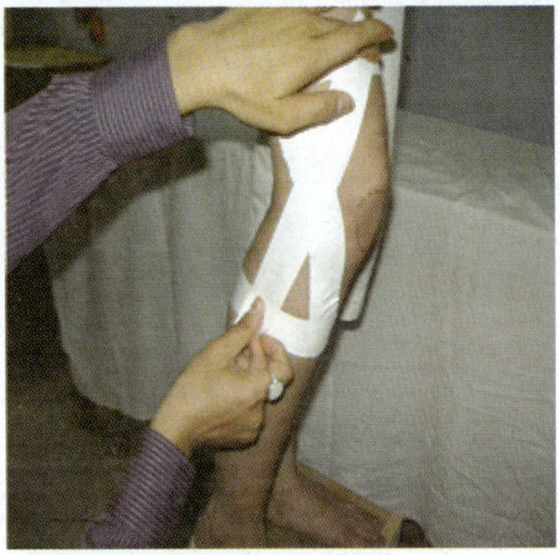

Fig. 5.10(a)

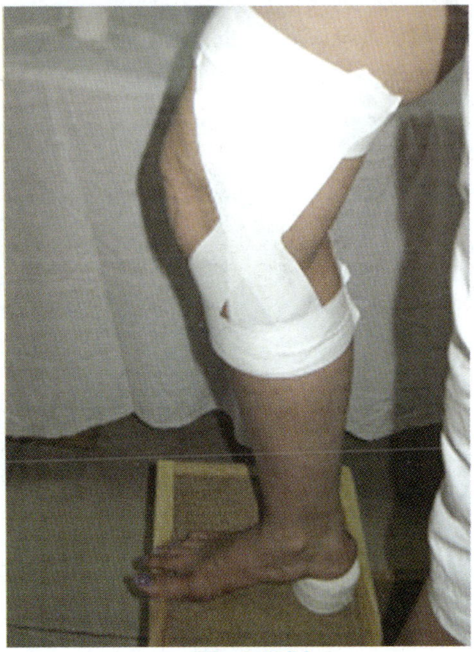

Fig. 5.10(b)

"BUTTERFLY" OR CHECK-REIN (Figs. 5.11 to 5.14)

Description: A combination of three or more vertical strips applied at angle of 10-15 degrees each other, placed at the axis of rotation of the joint to be taped. These strips can be of either non-elastic or elastic tape depending upon the injured structure and the goals of the taping.

Purpose: To restrict movement in more than a simple uniplanar direction, as so often found in normal motion. This "butterfly" or "check-rein" can resist stresses with inherent torsion components as well as those that are purely unidirectional.

Method: Steps in applying "butterfly" strips.

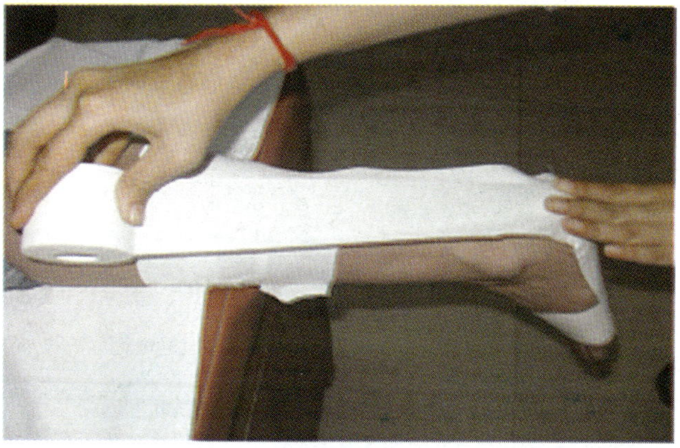

Fig. 5.11

FIRST STRIP: In a truly vertical position from the distal anchor to the proximal anchor.

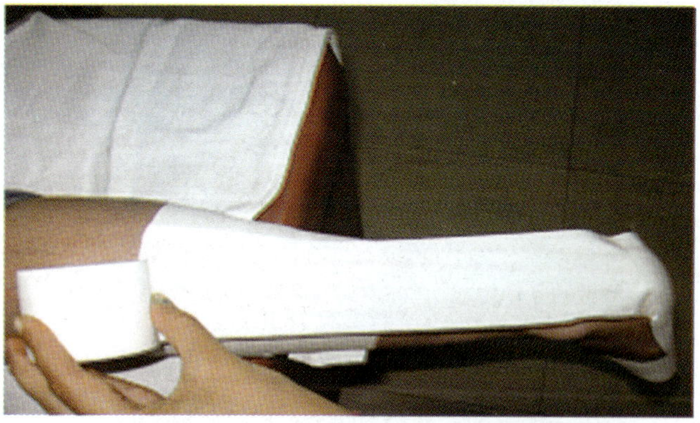

Fig. 5.12

SECOND STRIP: In a slightly rotated fashion in one direction.

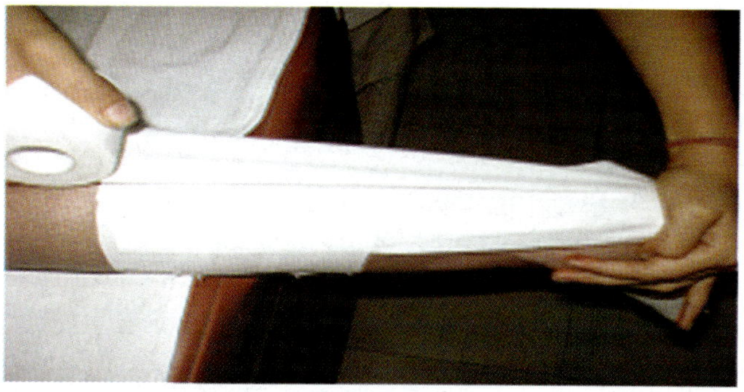

Fig. 5.13

THIRD STRIP: In a slightly rotated position opposite to the second strip.

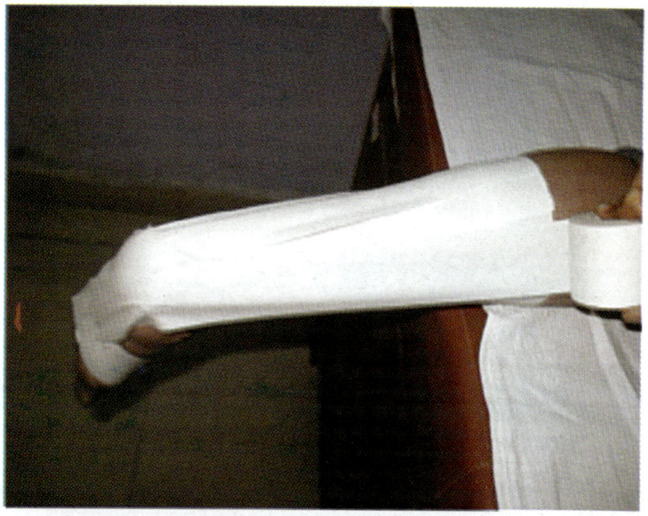

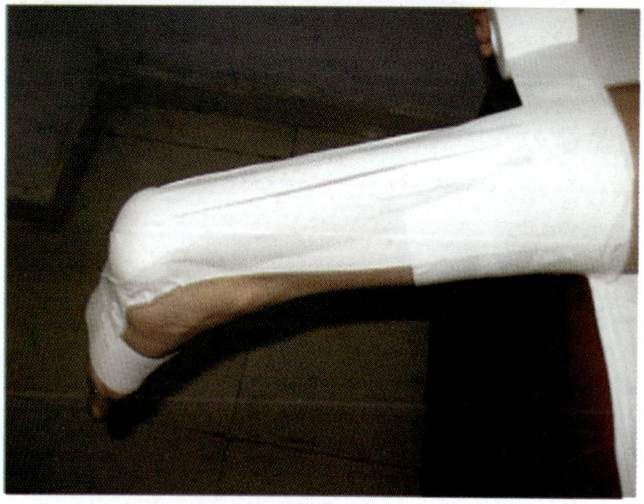

Fig. 5.14

FINAL STEP: Reanchor these strips.

NOTES:

- Proper poisoning of the injured limb is crucial to effective application.
- The axis of the three strips lies directly on joint line.

LOCKS (Figs. 5.15(a) to (c))

Description: A non elastic tape strip attached firmly to the underlying anchor reinforcing support.

Purpose: To reinforce joint stability yet allow protected, functional movements.

Methods: Strong tension is applied at key points in the application of the locking strip which reinforces the injured structure and stabilizes the joint.

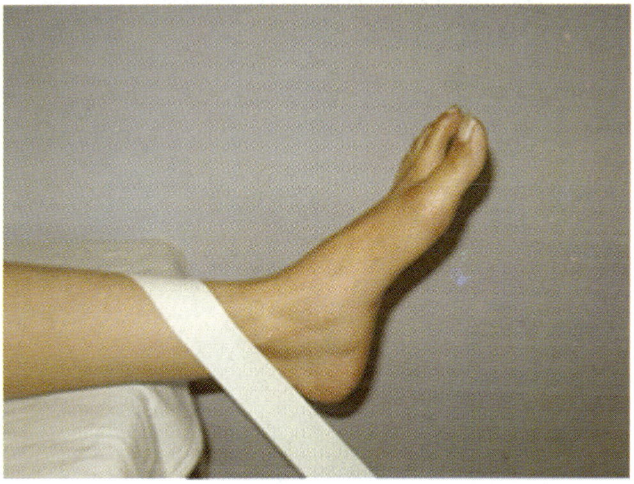

Fig. 5.15(a)

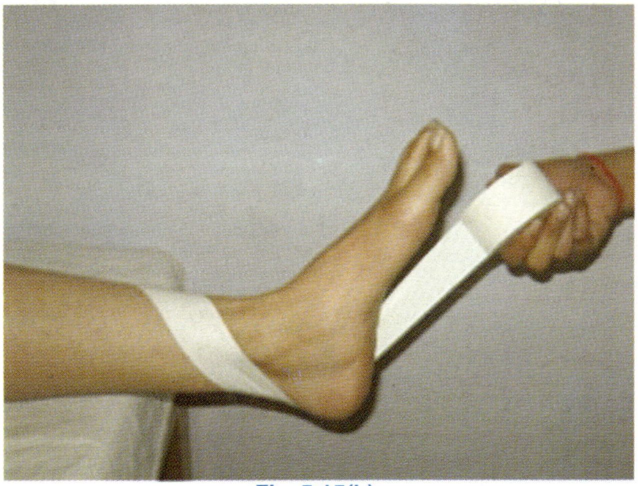

Fig. 5.15(b)

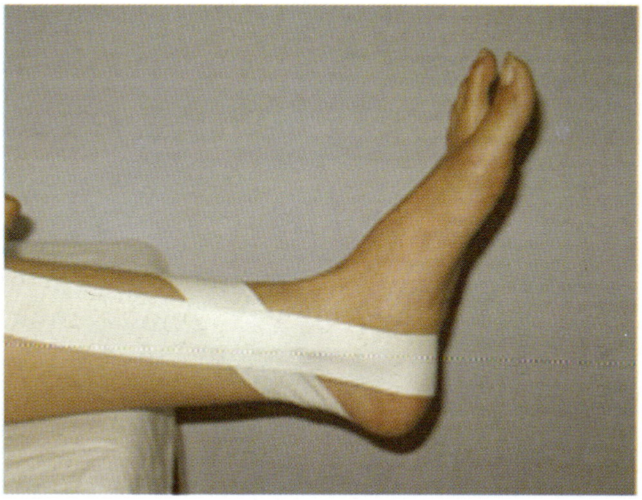

Fig. 5.15(c)

FIGURE OF 8 (Figs. 5.16(a) to (h))

Description: A strip of non elastic tape forming a Figure 8; usually applied as one of the last strips in an ankle or thumb taping.

Purpose: To give added stability; to cover any remaining open areas and/ or tape ends; to close the tape application neatly.

Method: Apply the tape by encircling one segment of the limb in one direction before crossing over to encircle the opposite segment in the opposite direction, thus forming a "Figure 8".

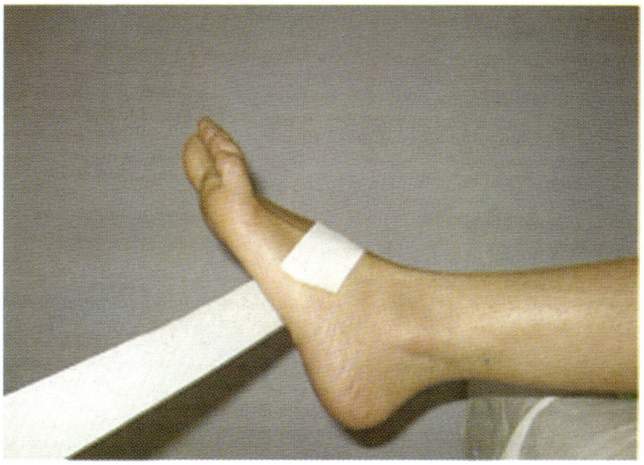

Fig. 5.16(a)

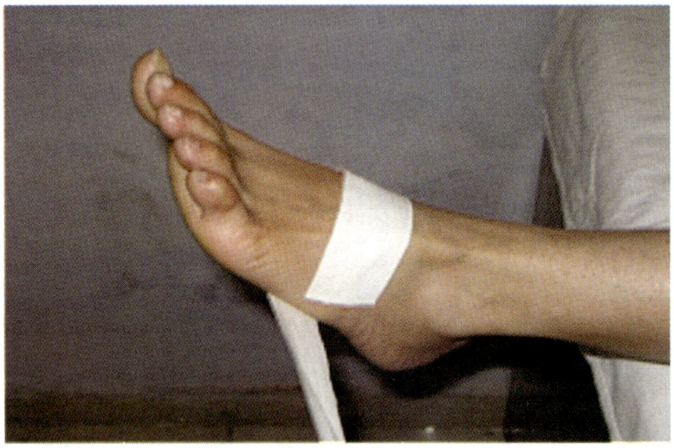

Fig. 5.16(b)

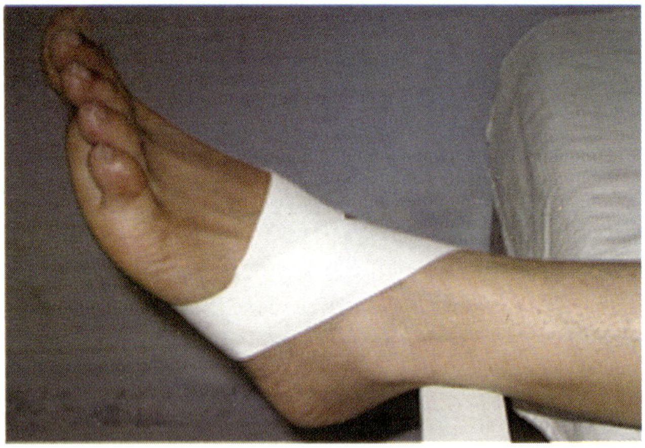

Fig. 5.16(c)

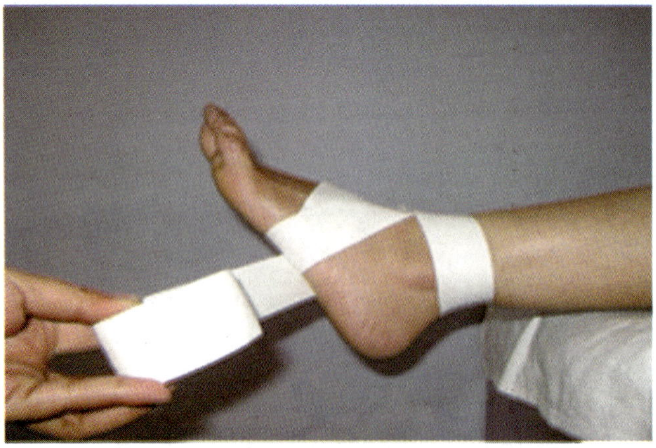

Fig. 5.16(d)

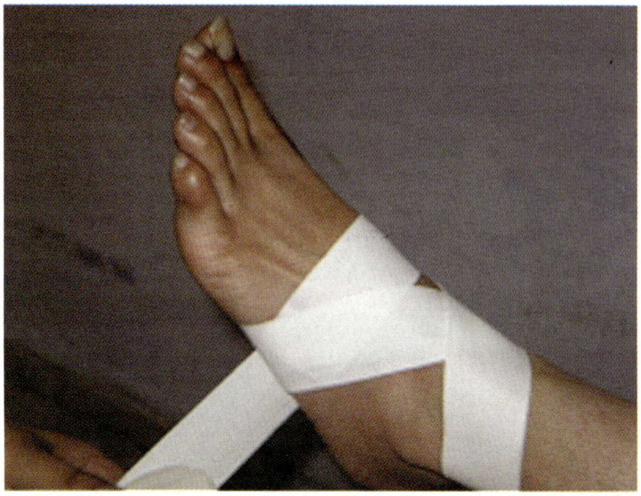

Fig. 5.16(e)

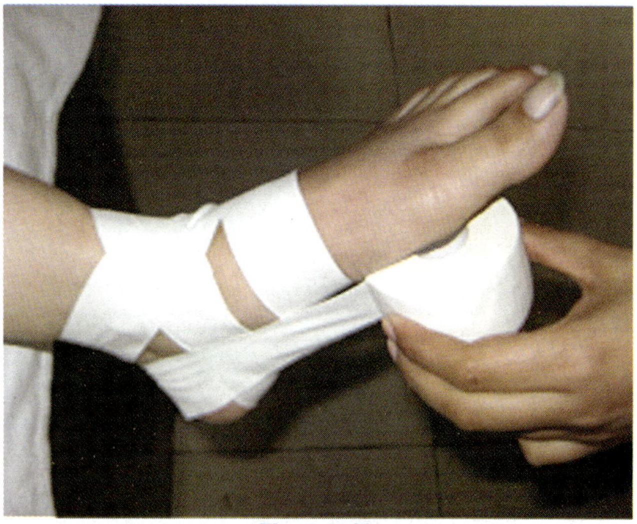

Fig. 5.16(f)

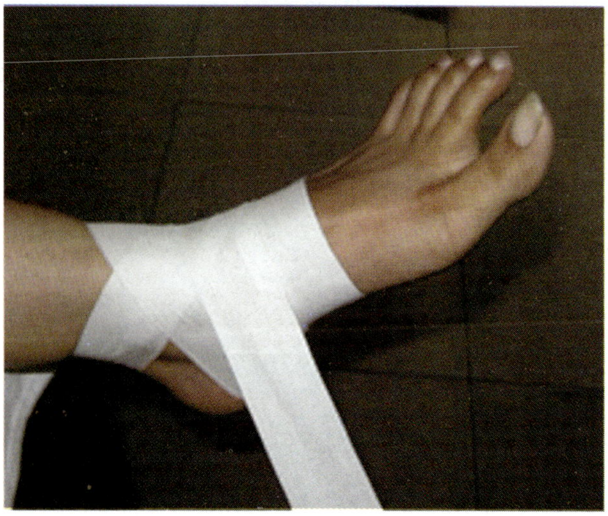

Fig. 5.16(g)

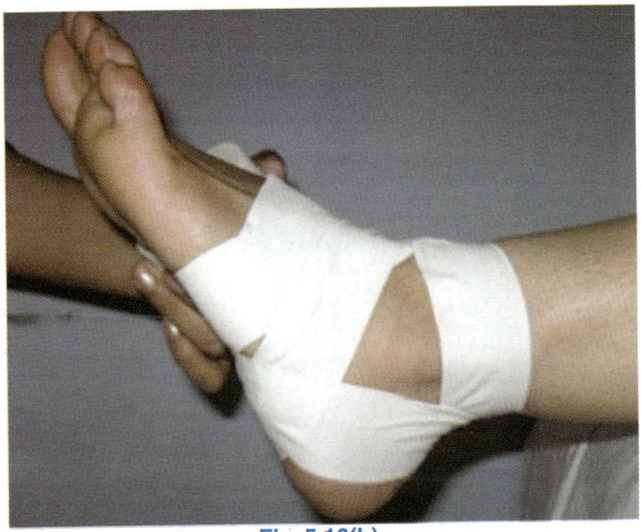

Fig. 5.16(h)

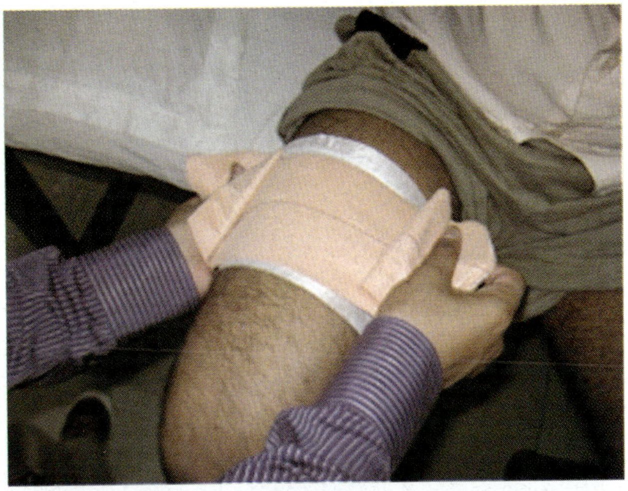

Fig. 5.17(a)

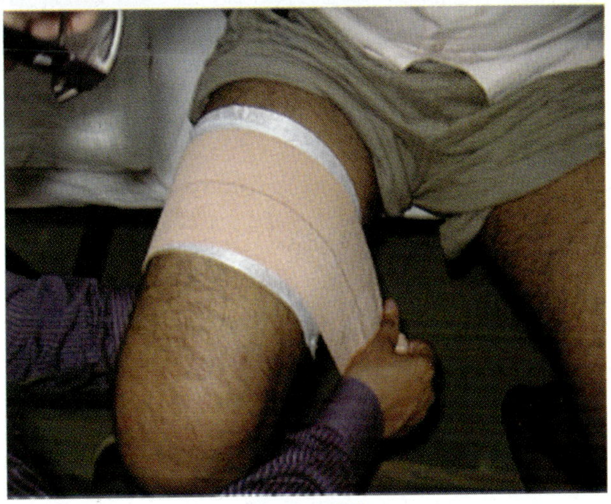

Fig. 5.17(b)

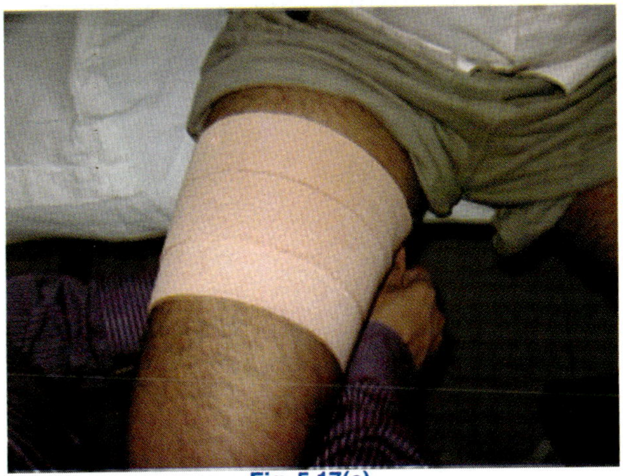

Fig. 5.17(c)

COMPRESSION STRIPS (5.17(a)-(d))

Description

Elastic adhesive tape strips applied with localized compression over a muscle injury.

Purpose

- To provide strong compressive forces localized to the injured area.
- To minimize subsequent swelling.
- To prevent further injury without compromising circulation.
- To permit activity.

Method

- Apply one layer of elastic adhesive tape directly to the skin with minimal tension to form a base.
- Apply pressure strip by holding the tape fully stretched while pressing firmly directly over the injury. Maintain the pressure while gradually releasing it behind the limb before overlapping the ends without tension to avoid a tourniquet effect. Repeat the compression strips with each overlapping the previous one by half until entire injured area-distal (lower) to proximal (upper) is covered.

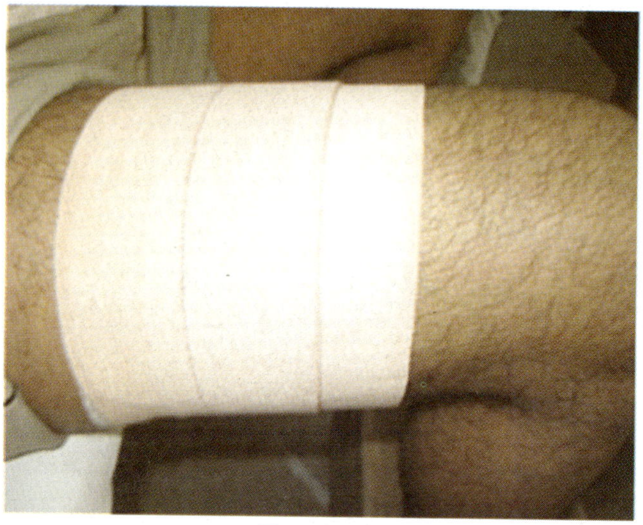

Fig. 5.17(d)

CLOSING-UP STRIPS (Figs. 5.18(a) to (b))

Description

Lightly place strips of either elastic or non-elastic tape which cover any remaining open areas or tape ends, nearly finishing the taping job.

Purpose

- To reduce the risk of skin blister by covering all open areas.
- To make the tape less likely to unwind during athletic activity.
- To give a neat appearance to the finished taping.

Method: Apply the strips of tape around the circumference of the limb, with a one-third to one-half width of overlap, starting proximally (upper end) and moving distally (lower end).

NOTE: By applying these strips from proximal to distal, the tape edges will not be pulled or rolled back when the athlete rapidly dresses for sport after taping.

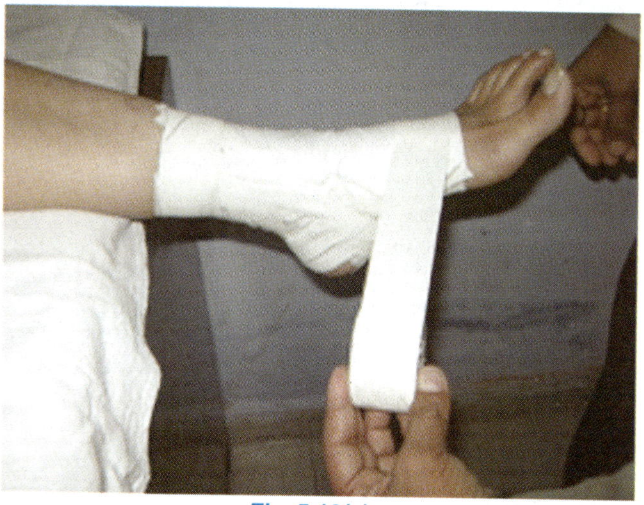

Fig. 5.18(a)

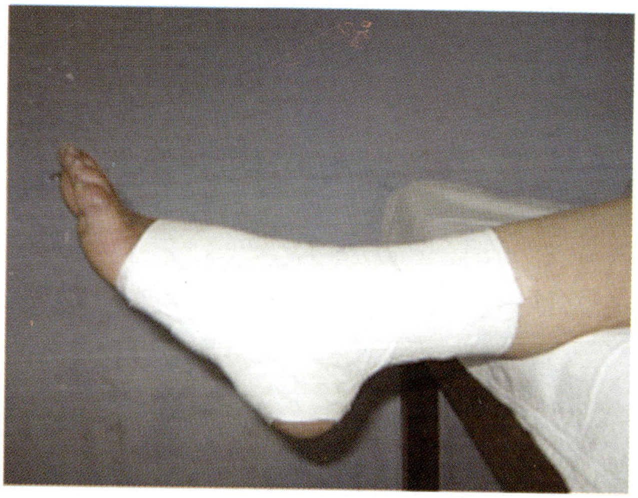

Fig. 5.18(b)

6 FOOT AND ANKLE TAPING

FOOT AND ANKLE

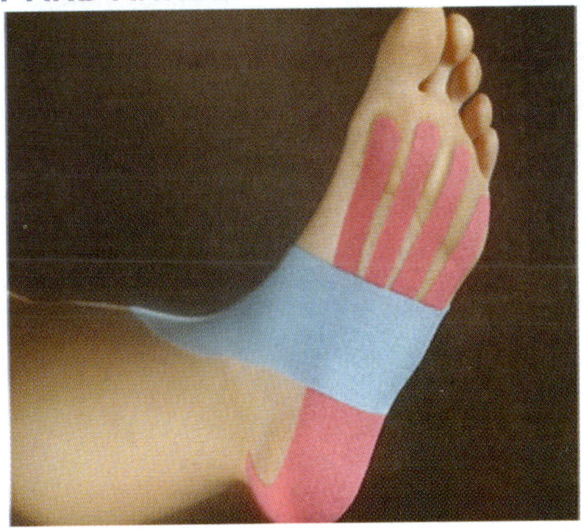

Fig. 6.1

The intent of taping is to provide protection while allowing functional movement thus preventing further damage to the injured structure or adjacent areas.

ANATOMICAL AREA: FOOT AND ANKLE

The articulation of foot and ankle are numerous and complex. The joint of the foot and curvature of the arches of the foot permit adaptation to irregular terrain. These joints offer suppleness and shock absorption through elasticity. This varied bony architecture and mobility predisposes to different types of injuries. Taped support can alleviate many stresses related to these conditions.

The **talo-crural** (the true ankle) joint is mainly responsible for dorsiflexion and plantar flexion while the **sub-talar joint** allows more lateral mobility–inversion and eversion–(sideways deviation) permitting the foot adapt to all angels of incline or slope. This relatively mobile **ankle joint** complex is dependent on numerous ligaments for its stability, and on tendons for its dynamic support. Forces through this relatively fragile joint make it vulnerable to stresses. The ankle is most easily injured during weight bearing activities which require quick changes of direction.

Right ankle and foot from the medial side and lateral side

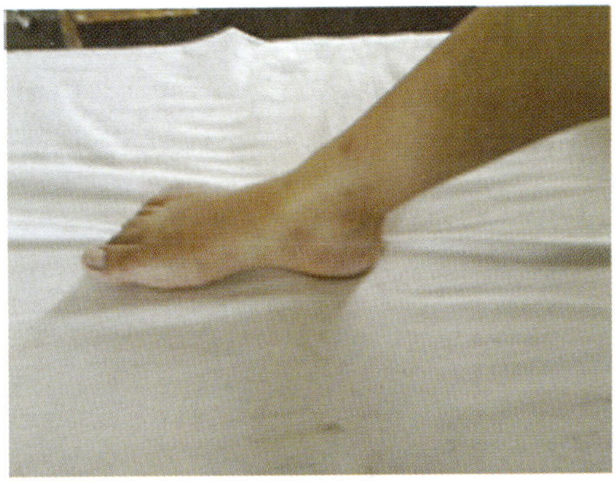

(a)

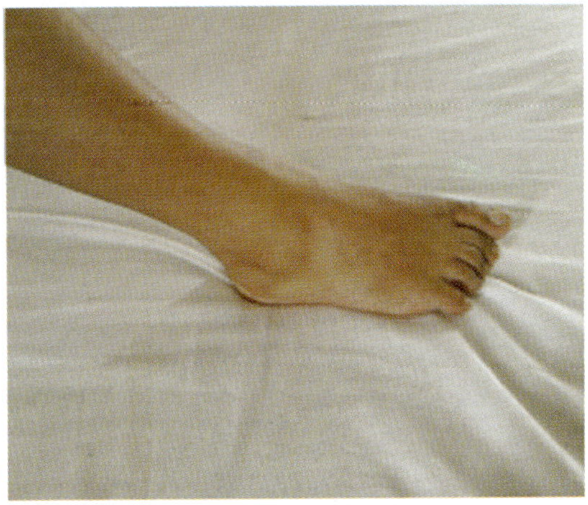

(b)

Fig. 6.2(a) and (b)

Right ankle and foot, from the lateral side: The most prominent surface features are the lateral malleolus the tendo calcaneus at the back and the tendon of Tibialis anterior at the front.

SURFACE ANATOMY OF BONES AND PALPATION OF SOFT TISSUES

1. Medial malleolus.
2. Tuberosity of navicular.

3. Lateral malleolus.
4. Tuberosity of calcaneus.
5. Tuberosity of base of 5 metatarsal.
6. Head of 5 metatarsal.
7. Sesamoid bone.

TENDONS

1. Tendo calcaneus.
2. Flexor hallucis longus.
3. Flexor digitorum longus.
4. Tibialis posterior.
5. Tibialis anterior.
6. Extensor hallucis longus.
7. Peroneus longus and brevis.
8. Extensor digitorum brevis.
9. Extensor digitorum longus.

ARTERIES

1. Dorsalis pedis.
2. Posterior tibialis.

VEINS

1. Great sapheneous.
2. Small sapheneous.

NERVES

1. Great sapheneous.
2. Posterior tibial.
3. Sural.

LIGAMENTS

1. Deltoid ligament.
   (a) Posterior tibiotalar part.
   (b) Tibiocalcanean part.
   (c) Anterior tibiotalar part.
2. Long plantar ligament.

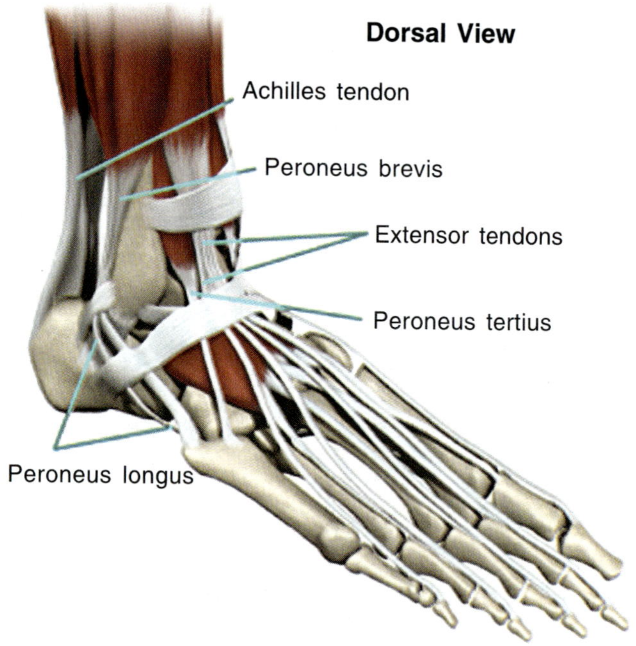

3. Anterior talofibular ligament.
4. Posterior talofibular ligament.
5. Tibio-fibular ligament.
6. Sustentaculum tali.
7. Tibio navicular part.
8. Calcaneo fibular ligament.
9. Anterior inferior tibiofibular ligament.
10. Posterior inferior tibiofibular ligament.
11. Talo navicular ligament.
12. Dorsal cuneonavicular ligament.
13. Dorsal tarso metatarsal ligament.
14. Dorsal metatarsal ligament.
15. Cervical ligament.
16. Dorsal calcaneo cuboid ligament.
17. Bifurcate (calcaneo cuboid and calcaneo navicular parts) ligament.

BONES

1. Calcaneus.
2. Medial malleolus of the tibia.

3. Groove for tibialis posterior tendon.
4. Lateral malleolus of tibia.
5. Groove for proneus brevis tendon.
6. Head of tibialis.
7. Trochlear surface of talar.
8. Groove for flexor hallucis longus tendon.
9. Tuberosity of navicular.
10. Tuberosity of base of 5th metatarsal.

TENDONS

1. Tibialis posterior.
2. Tibialis anterior.
3. Peroneus longus.
4. Flexor hallucis longus.

A variety of taping techniques are highly effective in supporting both ligamentous and musculo-tendinous conditions related to the ankle joint. With the application of proper taping technique, the athlete can rapidly resume normal competitive activity and/or intense training.

In this, details on the following items will prove useful:

- Specific purpose of each taping technique.
- Conditions appropriate for specific applications.
- A list of materials.
- Special notes.
- Positioning for taping procedure.
- Illustrated procedure.

TAPING FOR TOE SPRAIN

Purpose

- Support of first metatarsophalangeai (MTP) joint.
- Allows moderate flexion and some extension.
- Limits end range of flexion, extension and adduction.

Indication for use

- Sprain of first metatarsophalangeal (MTP) joint.
- For a medial collateral ligament sprain: Abduct the toe and reinforce the medial restraining tape strip.
- For a plantar ligament sprain (hyper-extension injury): Reinforce the tape on the plantar surface to limit extension.
- For a lateral collateral ligament sprain: Reinforce with buddy taping to the first toe (**for an example of buddy taping used with figure).**
- For a dorsal capsular sprain (hyper flexion): Reinforce the tape on the dorsal surface to limit flexion.
- Hyper flexion to the first MTP joint: "turf toe".
- Contusion of first MTP joint: "jammed toe", "stubbed toe".
- Painful bunions.

NOTES:

- The base of the fifth metatarsal bone is a sensitive, vulnerable area prone to pressure pain and blister if tape is tight.
- To avoid constriction, minimal tension must be used when wrapping circumference anchors.
- Application of lubricant to adjacent toes and/or the inside of the toe box of the shoe will prevent rubbing.
- Trimming toe nails will lessen the risk of irritation.
- Careful application of minimal amount of tape is particularly important when taping for sports when required tight-fitting shoes or boots.

MATERIALS

Razor.

Skin toughener spray.

(3/4 inch) White tape or (split 1.5 inch tape).

INJURY: TOE SPRAIN

TERMINOLOGY

- Sprain of medial or lateral collateral ligament.
- Hyper flexion with capsular injury.
- Hyperextension with capsular injury.
- Sprain of the planter ligament.
- "Jammed" toe; "stubbed" toe; "turf" toe.

ETIOLOGY

- Sudden forced flexion, extension or abduction.
- Sudden longitudinal impact against a hard surface.
- Repetitive dorsiflexion of great toe.
- Chronic sprain.
- Inadequately supportive footwear on artificial turf.

SYMPTOMS

- Tenderness of the first metatarsophalangeal joint.
- Often swollen.
- Active movement testing.
  a. Pain on end range flexion with hyper flexion injuries.
  b. Pain on end range extension with hyperextension injuries.
  c. Pain on end range abduction with medial collateral ligament sprain.
- Passive movement testing.
  a. Pain on end range flexion with hyper flexion injuries.
  b. Pain on end range abduction with medial collateral ligament.
  c. Pain on end range abduction with medial collateral ligament sprain.
- Resistance testing in (neutral position): No significant pain on moderate resistance.
- Stress testing.
  a. Pain with or without laxity on medial (or lateral) stress with 1st and 2nd degree sprains of the medial (or lateral) collateral ligaments.
  b. Instability with less pain in 3rd degree sprains.

TREATMENT

Early

- R.I.C.E.S.
- Taping for toe sprain.
- Therapeutic modalities.

Later

Continued physiotherapy including:

- Therapeutic modalities.
- Passive mobilizations if painful stiff.
- Flexibility.
- Strengthening exercises.
- Gradual pain free reintegration to sports activities with taped support.
- A shoe with stiff soles for reinforcement may be necessary.
- Dynamic weight bearing activity should start only after 45 degree of pain free dorsiflexion is attained.

SEQUELAE

- Pain.
- Chronic swelling.
- Diminished mobility.
- Weakness.
- Chronic synovitis.
- Flexor hallucis longus tendinitis.
- Degenerate changes leading to hallux rigidus (stiff first toe).

POSITIONING (Fig. 6.3(a))

Sitting on the treatment table with the injured foot slightly overhanging the end of table.

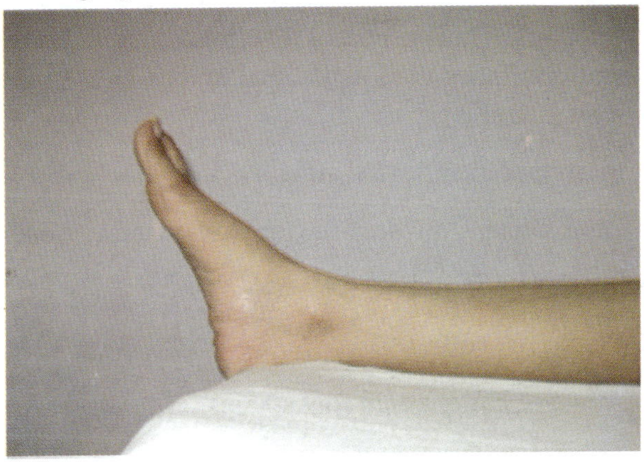

Fig. 6.3(a)

PROCEDURE

1. Clean the area and shave the dorsum of foot if hairy.
2. Spray area with skin toughener or quick dry adhesive spray to ensure adherence.
3. Place an anchor of 2 cm of white tape around the distal toe at base of toe nail.
4. Place two anchors of white tape around in step and arch of foot (Fig. 6.3(b)).

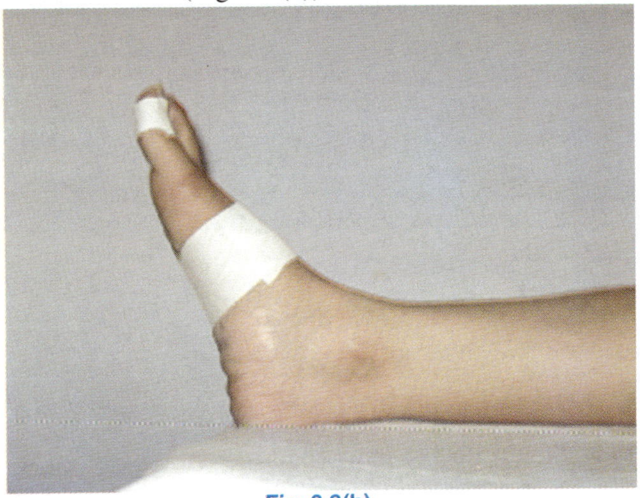

Fig. 6.3(b)

5. Place a longitudinal supporting strip of 2 cm of white tape from distal to proximal anchor on medial aspect of foot (Fig. 6.3(c)).

NOTE:

Abduct the toe slightly and apply two strip with tension when taping for medial collateral ligament sprain or bunions.

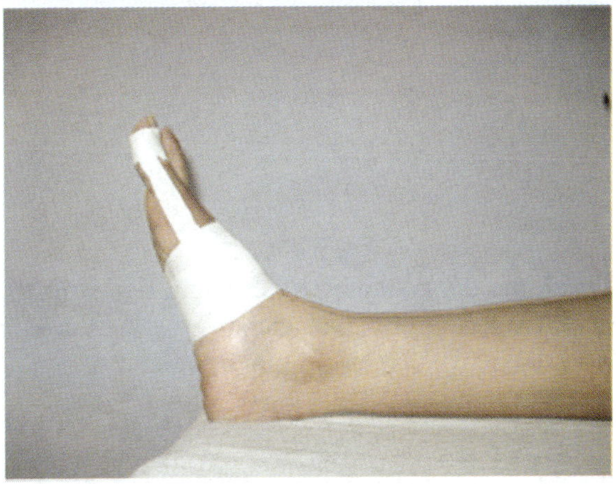

Fig. 6.3(c)

6. Cross this with second strip with medial aspect of distal anchor crossing MTP joint at its midpoint on plantar aspect(Fig. 6.3(d)).

NOTE:

Extension must be adequately limited with the tape when taping hyperextension injuries.

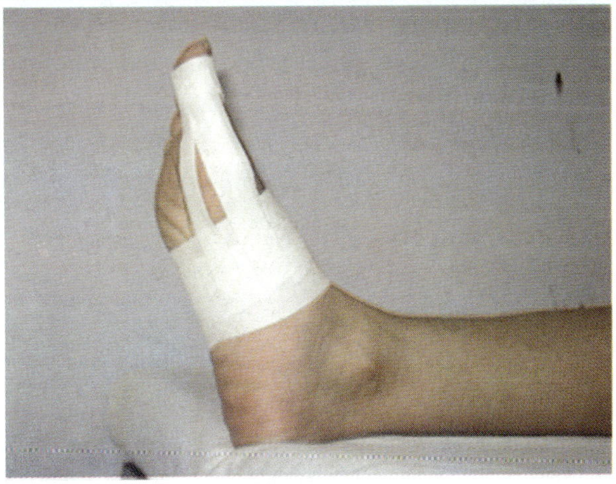

Fig. 6.3(d)

7. Begin dorsal taping with a 2 cm strip from the medial aspect of the distal anchor to dorsal aspect of the proximal anchor (Fig. 6.3(e)).

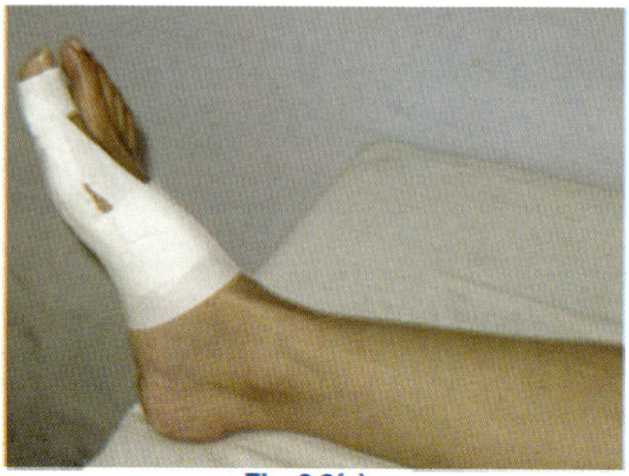

Fig. 6.3(e)

8. Finish the dorsal taping by crossing this strip from lateral aspect of proximal anchor, crossing the taping over dorsal MPT joint (Fig. 6.3(f)).

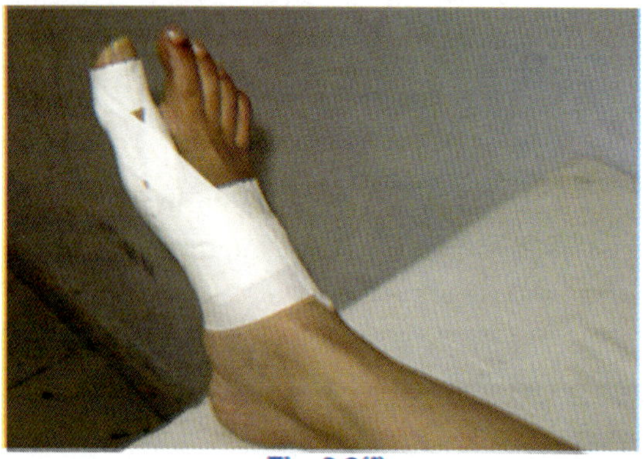

Fig. 6.3(f)

9. Close up taping with light circumferential strips covering sites of original anchors starting proximally and moving distally, overlapping each previous strip (Fig. 6.3(g)).

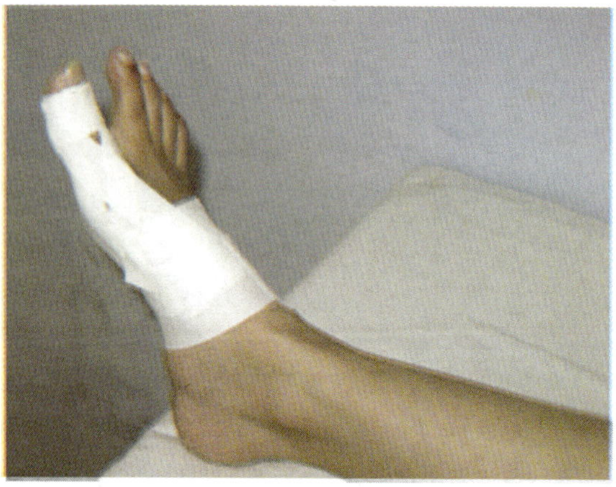

Fig. 6.3(g)

10. Test taping for adequate restriction to ensure adequate pain free functional support.

TAPING FOR LONGITUDINAL ARCH SPRAIN (Fig. 6.4(a))

Purpose

- Supports plantar aspect of foot (functionally shortens and reinforces the longitudinal arches medial more than lateral).
- Permits plantar flexion mobility.
- Limits extension (dorsiflexion) of mid tarsal joints.

Indications for use

- Plantar fasciitis.
- Acute or chronic mid foot sprains.
- Flat feet or fallen arches.
- Medial knee pain caused by flat feet.
- Bony spurs.
- Shin splints.

NOTES:

- Pressure on base of 5th metatarsal bone can cause acute pain.
- Pressure on its neighbouring artery can cause pain and compromise circulation.
- Tape thickness must be kept to a minimum for sports requiring a tight-fitting boot or shoes.
- Excessive medial tension must be avoided, particularly in ankles predisposed to inversion sprains.

Materials

- Razor.
- Skin toughener spray.
- 1 /1.5 inch white tape.

TERMINOLOGY

- Chronic or acute inflammation of plantar fascia.
- Heel spurs.

ETIOLOGY

- Intrinsically tight plantar fascia.

- Poor foot biomechanics.
- Sudden change in training routine: i.e. distance, frequency, speed, change of terrain.
- Poorly supportive or new footwear.
- Secondary to midfoot sprain or tarsal hypo mobility.

SYMPTOMS

- Pain and tenderness on plantar aspect of foot: More concerned on the medial aspect of calcaneal attachment.
- Active movement testing: No significant pain in non-weightbearing position.
- Passive movement testing: Pain on full stretch of fascia.
- Resistance testing.
- Pain on first steps after resting.

TREATMENT

Physiotherapy including:

- R.I.C.E.S.
- Therapeutic modalities (use of laser or ultrasound can be particularly helpful).
- Support: Taping: **LONGITUDINAL ARCH TAPING.**
- Rest: Reduction of weight bearing activities.
- Selective stretching of tendo-Achilles and of plantar fascia.
- Strengthening of plantar muscles.
- Heel lifts can be helpful in acute phase.

SEQUELAE

- Injury often becomes chronic without correct treatment.
- Development of heel spurs.
- Tight tendo-achillies complex.
- May predispose to shin splints.

POSITIONING (Figs. 6.4(a) to (h))

Either prone lying with knee slightly bent (as illustrated) or sitting up facing the taper.

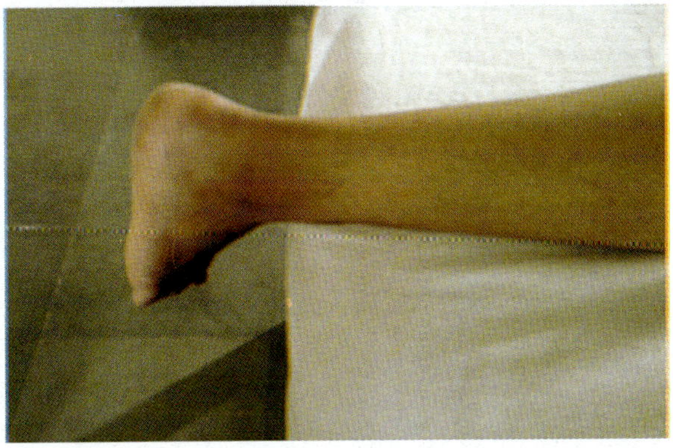

Fig. 6.4(a)

PROCEDURE

1. Clean foot and check for skin infections or skin conditions and signs of chronic inflammatory diseases.
2. Shave dorsum of foot if excessively hairy.
3. Spray area with skin toughener.

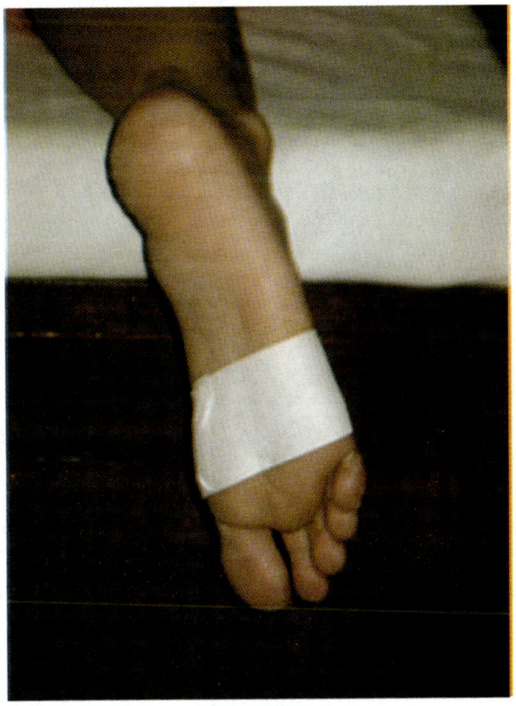

Fig. 6.4(b)

4. Place anchor strips of using light tension around the foot at the level of the heads of metatarsals.

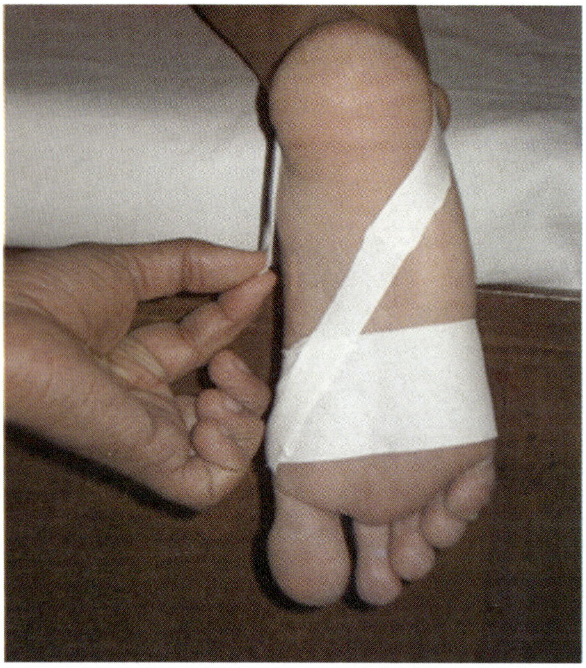

Fig. 6.4(c)

5. Using firm tension, place a strip of less width tape from the head of the first metatarsal under the arch around the heel.
6. Finish at the medial aspect of the first metatarsal, shortening medial arch.

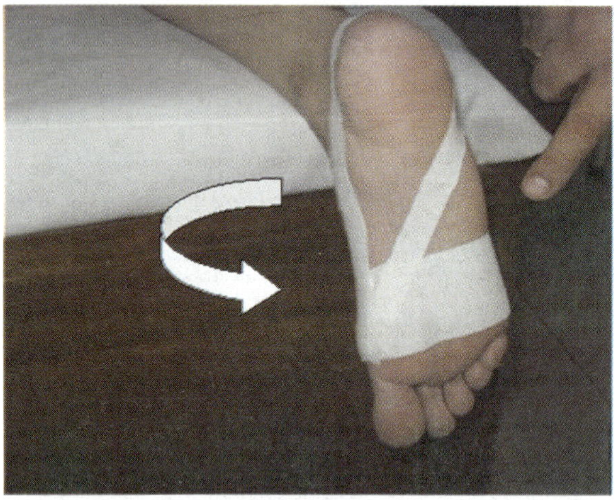

Fig. 6.4(d)

7. Starting from the lateral aspect of the anchor's plantar surface, apply a second strip, with strong tension, crossing the transverse arch diagonally around the heel.

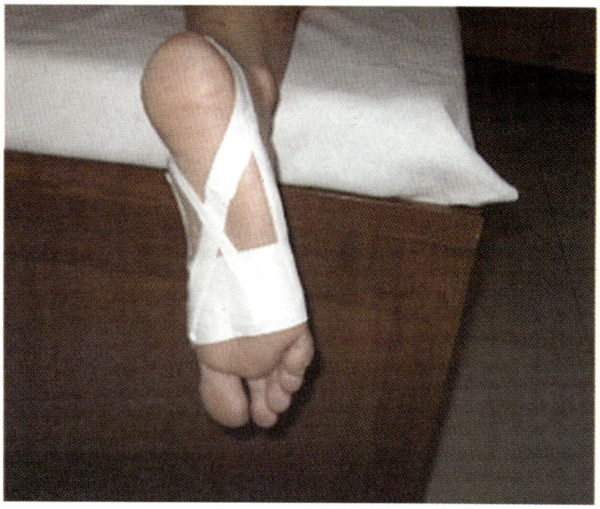

Fig. 6.4(e)

8. Pass behind the heel without tension and finish over the lateral aspect of the head of the fifth metatarsal.

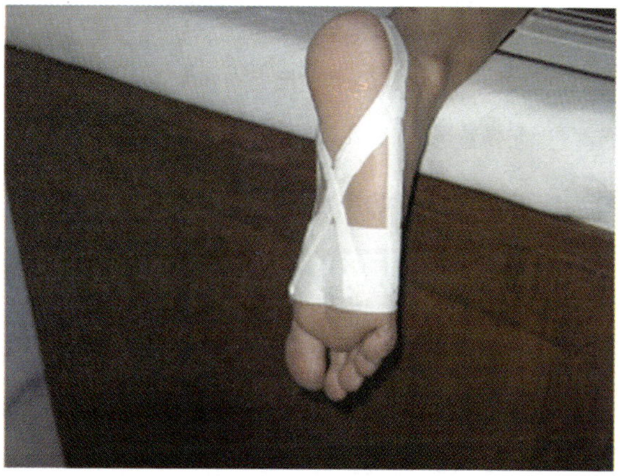

Fig. 6.4(f)

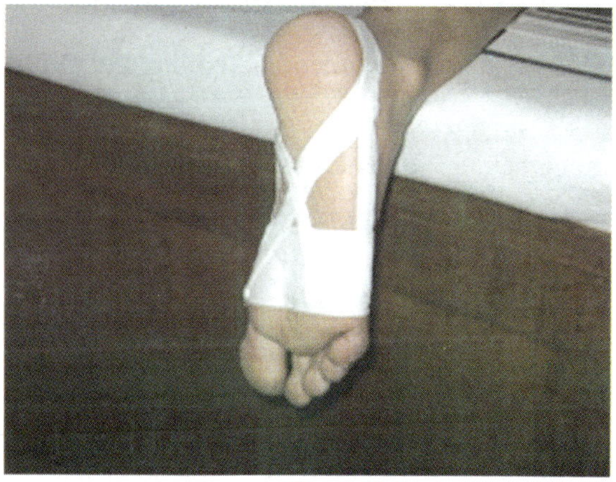

Fig. 6.4(g)

9. Apply reinforcement strips in the same way.

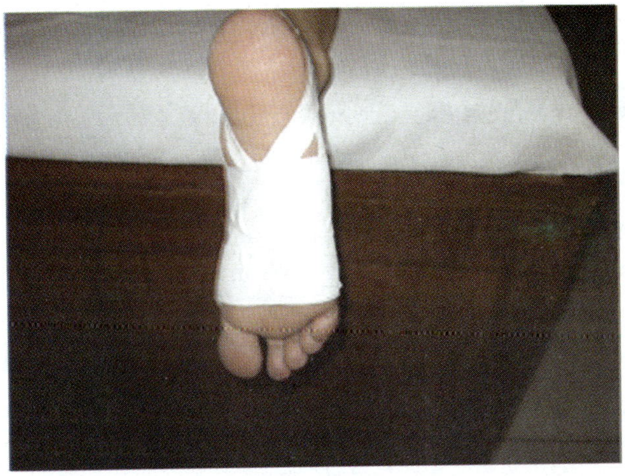

Fig. 6.4(h)

10. Close up with circumferential strips apply with firm upward pressure, following contours of foot with each strip, beginning at the heads of the metatarsals, progressing towards the heel.

Check the degree of support. There should be significant or complete reduction of pain on weightbearing.

TAPING FOR LATERAL ANKLE SPRAIN

Purpose

- Offers lateral stability with specific reinforcement.
- Prevents inversion.
- Restricts end range plantar flexion and some eversion.
- Allows almost full dorsiflexion and functional plantar flexion.

Indications for use

- Lateral ankle sprain (inversion sprain).
- Injuries of the calcaneo-fibular and the anterior talo-fibular ligaments, in combination, the most commonly injured.
- For medial ankle sprains (deltoid ligament): Use a horseshoe instead of a " j" shape.

MATERIALS

- Razor.
- Skin toughener spray.
- Prowrap.
- (1.5 in.) white tape.
- (3/4 inch) felt or foam cut into horseshoe or "j" shape.
- (3/4 inch) felt heel lift.
- (3 inch) elastic wrap for small ankles.
- (4 inch) for large ankles.

TAPING IS ADAPTED THROUGHOUT THE PROGRESSIVE REHABILITATION HEALING STAGE:

1. **SUBACUTE STAGE**: (After 48 hours post injury) support with felt J and heel lift while beginning to weight bear.
2. **FUNCTIONAL STAGE**: Specific ligamentous support with reinforcement of stability for moderate to dynamic activity.
3. **RETURN TO SPORT STAGE**: Reintegration with support adapted to specific sports requirements ranging from training to competition.

LATERAL ANKLE SPRAIN (TYPICALLY A COMBINATION OF TWO LIGAMENTS CALCANEO-FIBULAR AND ANTERIOR TALO-FIBULAR)

TERMINOLOGY

- Inversion sprain.
- "Turned" ankle.

ETIOLOGY

- Forced inversion with plantar flexion.
- "rolling –over" on ankle.
- Often secondary to inadequate rehabilitation of a pervious ankle sprain (reduced proprioception).
- The most commonly injured combination of ankle ligaments.

SYMPTOMS

- Local pain, swelling, discolouration and tenderness anteriorly and inferior to the lateral malleolus.

- Active movement testing: Pain on plantar flexion with inversion.
- Resistance testing (neutral position): No significant pattern of pain with moderate resistance.
- Stress testing:
  a. Pain, with or without laxity, on anterior "drawer" test (forward gliding of the talus under the tibio-fibular mortice) indicates a 1st or 2nd degree sprain of the anterior talo-fibular ligament.
  b. Instability on forward displacement of talus away from the lateral malleolus indicates a 3rd degree sprain of the same ligament .
  c. Pain with or without some laxity on talar tilt test indicates a 1st or 2nd degree sprain of the fibula-calcaneal.
  d. Instability or "opening up" on the talar tilt test (often with little or no pain) indicative of a 3rd degree sprain of this ligament.

TREATMENT

Early

- R.I.C.E.S.
- Taping 1st 48 hours (acute ankle injury).
- Therapeutic modalities.

Later

Continued physiotherapy including:

- Therapeutic modalities.
- Transverse friction massage.
- Modified fitness activities.
- Progressive pain-free rehabilitation including:
  a. Range of motion.
  b. Flexibility.
  c. Strength: Non-weight bearing to weight bearing.
  d. Proprioception.
- Gradual pain-free reintegration to sports activity with specific taping.
- Prevention of recurrent sprains.

SEQUELAE

- Anterior talo-crural and sub-talar instability if ligaments are not supported in a shortened position during healing phase.
- Weakness and/or tendinitis of peroneal muscles.
- Extensor digitorum longus is often injured simultaneously predisposing to chronic residual weakness.
- Reduced proprioception.
- Repeated injury caused by poor proprioception and joint instability.
- Chronic swelling in the sinus tarsi and around the tip of the lateral malleolus.

POSITIONING (Figs. 6.5(a) to (u))

Lying supine or long sitting support at mid calf with the foot off the end of the table. The ankle must be held at a 90 degree angle throughout the taping.

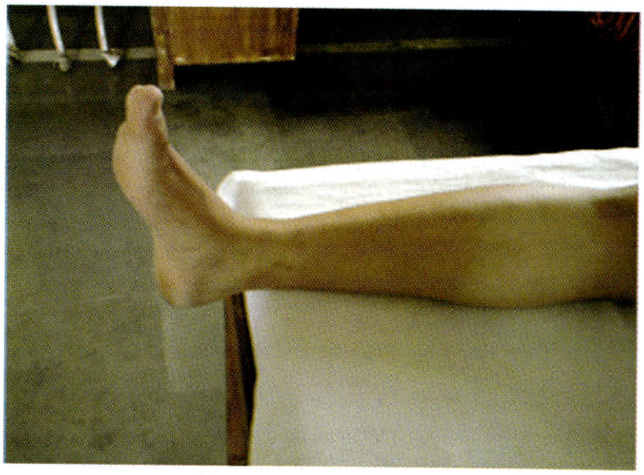

Fig. 6.5(a)

PROCEDURE

1. Ensure that the area to be taped is clean, shaved and dry.

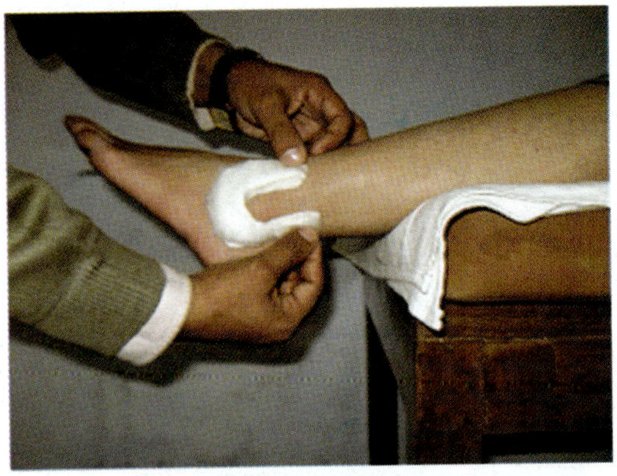

Fig. 6.5(b)

2. To control swelling cut a felt or dense foam pad in the shape of a "U" or a horseshoe to fill the hollows around the malleolus (ankle bone). Bevel the edges of the pad to form fit all the contours (Fig. 6.5(b)).
3. Check skin for cuts, blisters or irritated areas before spraying with skin toughener.

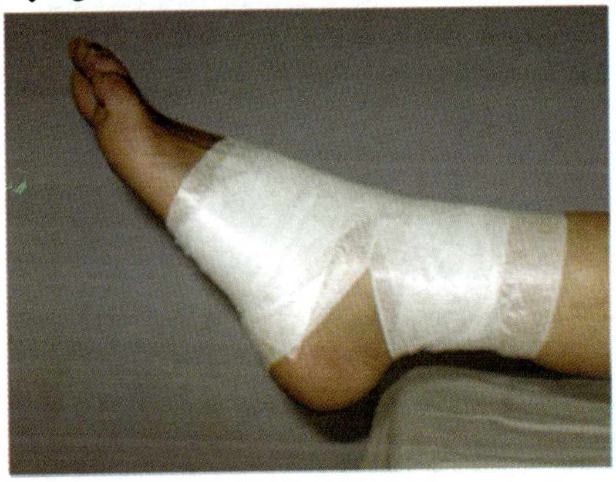

Fig. 6.5(c)

4. Apply prowrap to area to be taped.

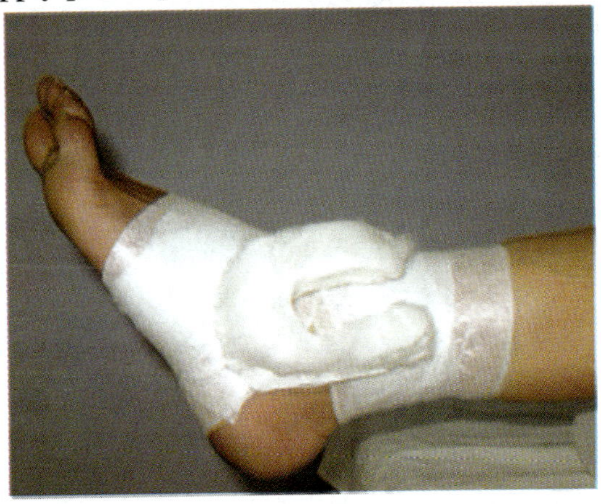

Fig. 6.5(d)

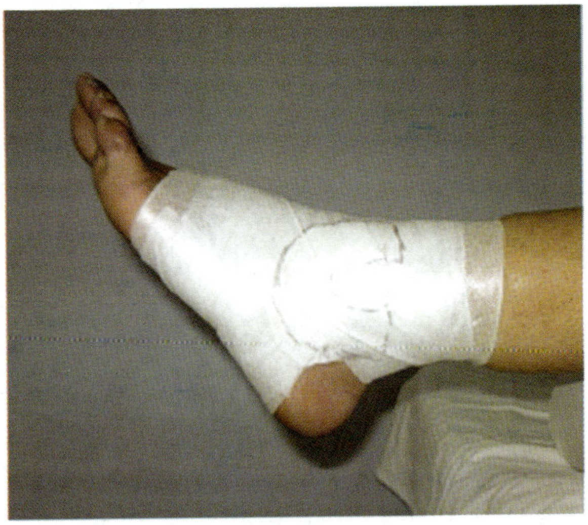

Fig. 6.5(e)

5. Attach the felt piece with a figure-8 of prowrap.
6. Using light tension, apply two overlapping, circumferential anchor strips of 3.8 cm (1.5 inch). White tape below the calf bulk at the musculo-tendinous junction.

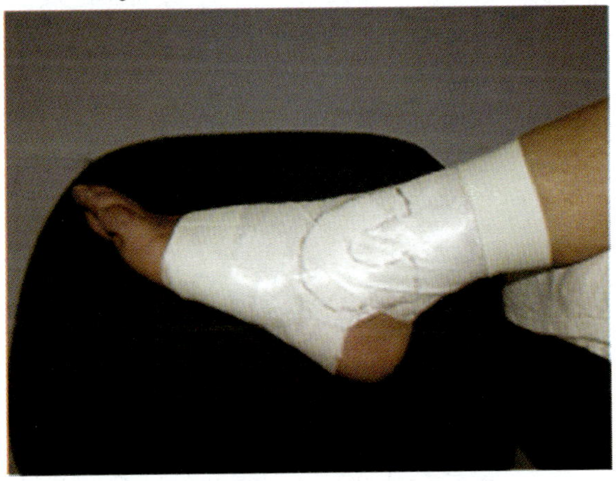

Fig. 6.5(f)

7. Apply two overlapping anchor strips around the forefoot.

Tips: Allow for some splaying of metatarsals to avoid discomfort when subjected to weight bearing.

NOTE: These anchors must be in direct contact with the skin to ensure support.

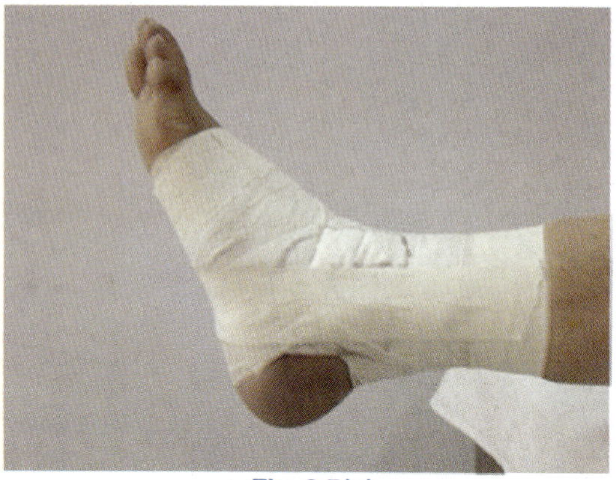

Fig. 6.5(g)

8. Apply a stirrup of starting from the upper anchor medially. Cover the posterior edge of the medial malleolus. Pass beneath the heel, and up, covering the posterior edge of the malleolus pull up strongly to apply specific tension over the lateral side and affix the tape to the upper anchor laterally.

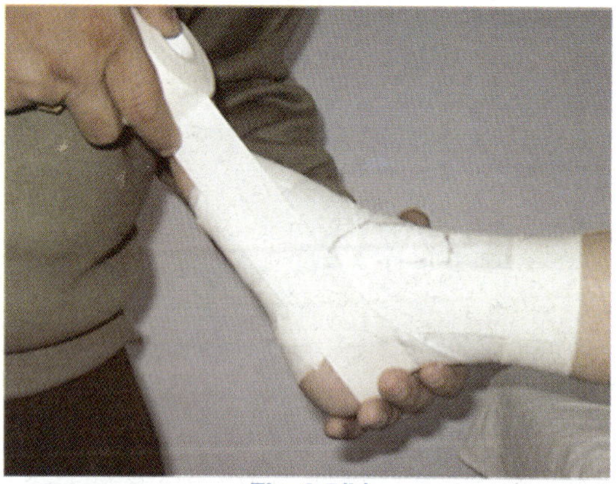

Fig. 6.5(h)

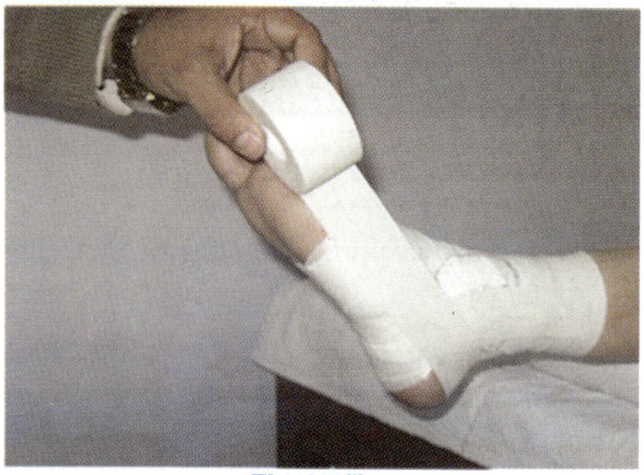

Fig. 6.5(i)

9. Starting on the medial side of the distal anchor, apply a horizontal strip passing behind the heel and covering the tip of the lateral malleolus. Put extra tension on the lateral side before reattaching the tape to the distal anchor on its lateral side.

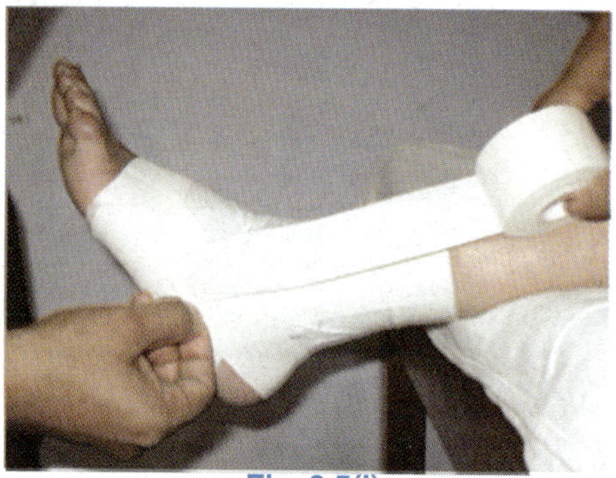

Fig. 6.5(j)

10. Apply reinforcement on the medial side, overlapping the previous stirrup by 2/3, anteriorly.

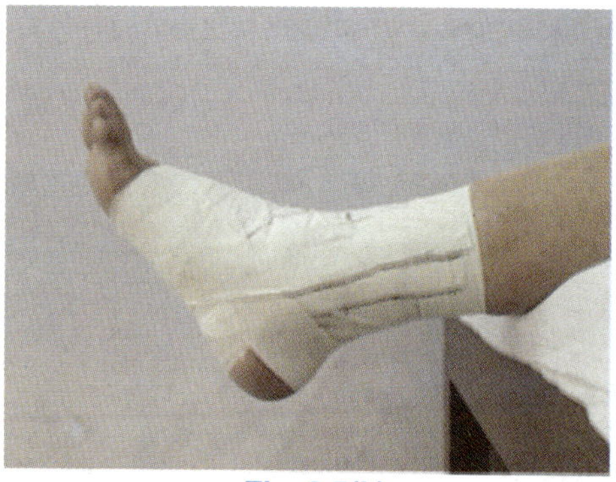

Fig. 6.5(k)

11. Apply a reinforcement horizontal on the lateral, overlapping the previous strip covering malleoli.

12. We can always apply a third reinforcement on the medial side overlapping the previous by 2/3 anteriorly providing more stability.

NOTES:

- A third horizontal strip may be necessary when taping large feet and when additional horizontal stability is required .
- These stirrups may be "fanned" when the athlete is at the returning to sport stage of rehabilitation.

13. Repeat the proximal and distal anchors.

14. Apply the first lateral ankle lock.

    a.. Begin on the anterior shin passing towards the lateral aspect of the ankle.

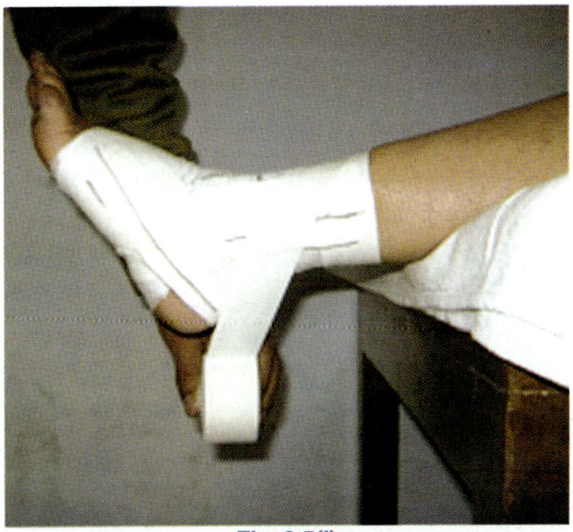

Fig. 6.5(l)

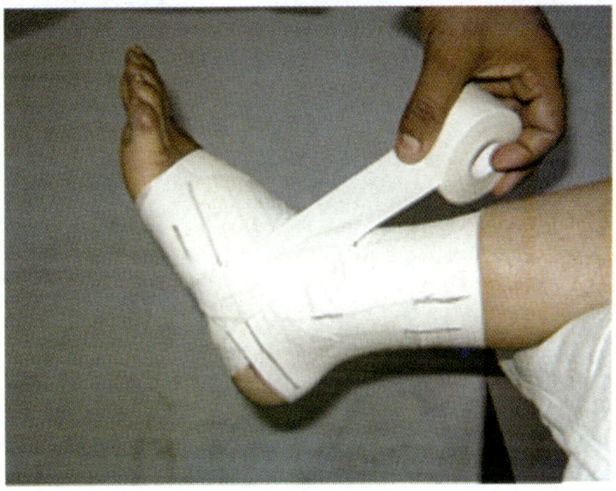

Fig. 6.5(m)

b. Continue behind the Achilles tendon, around and under the heel.

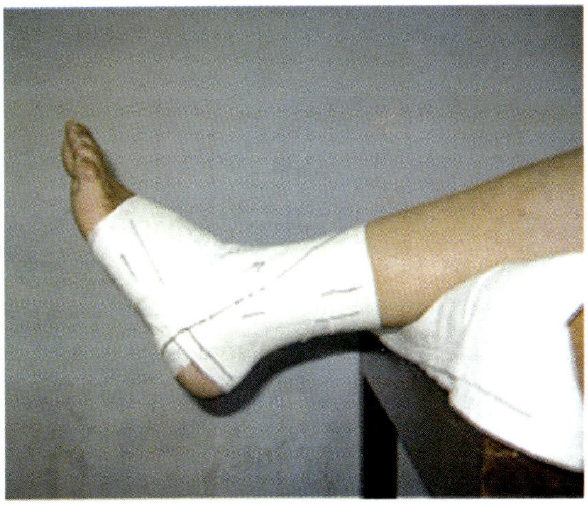

Fig. 6.5(n)

c. Then apply strong tension up over the lateral side to the lateral upper anchor.

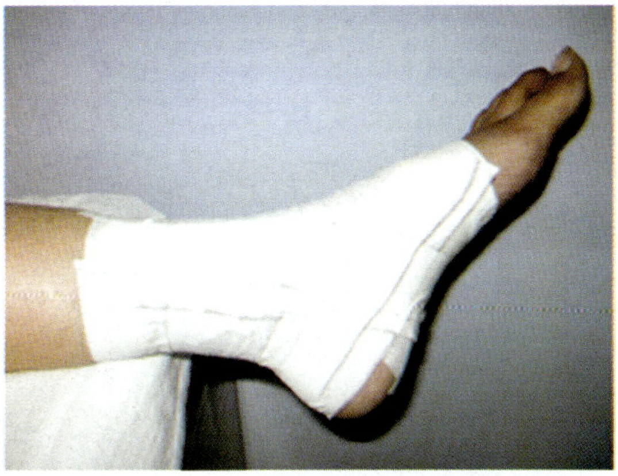

Fig. 6.5(o)

15. Repeat the ankle lock on lateral side overlapping the previous strip.

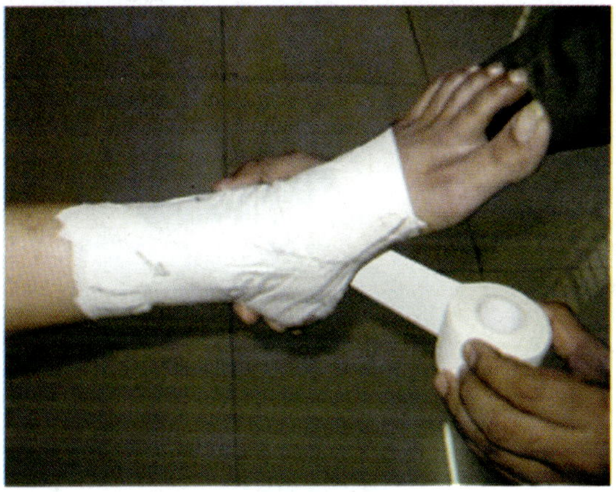

Fig. 6.5(p)

16. To balance stability apply the ankle lock once on the medial side with less tension when pulling up on the medial side.

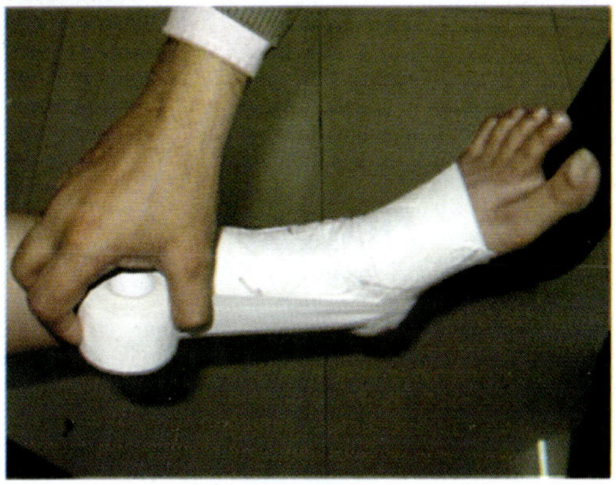

Fig. 6.5(q)

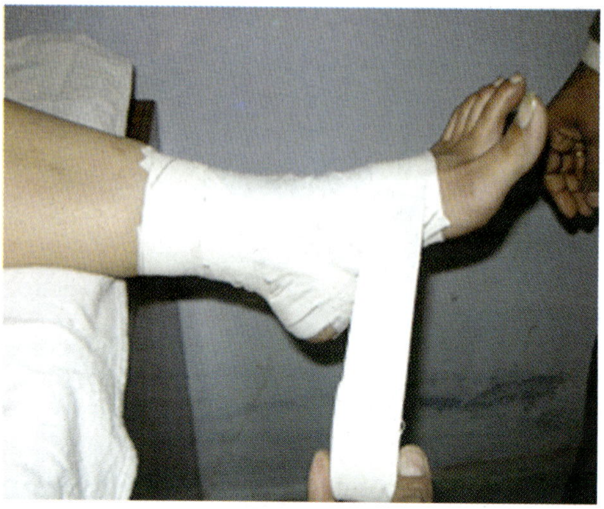

Fig. 6.5(r)

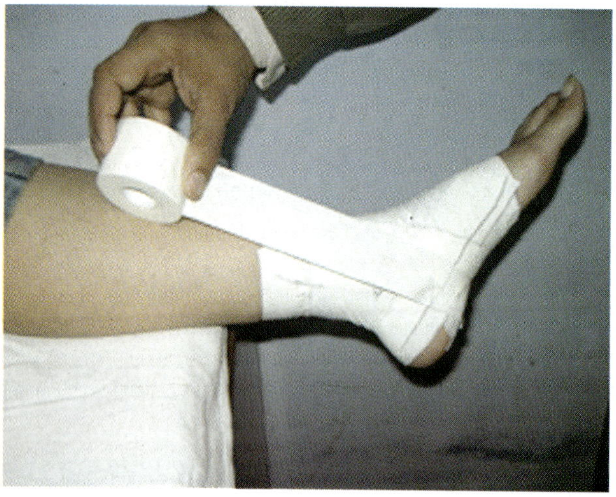

Fig. 6.5(s)

18. Reanchor proximally.

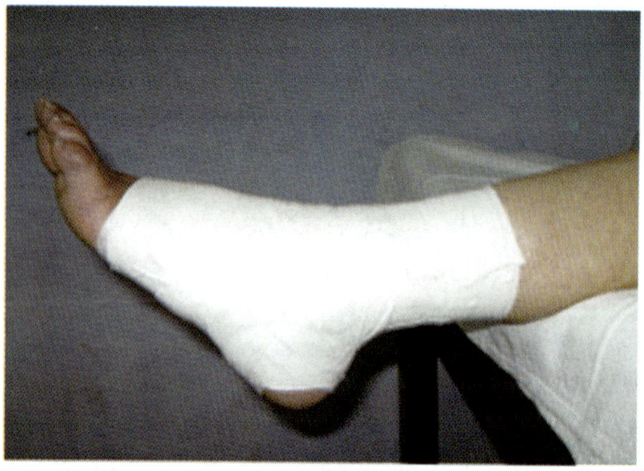

Fig. 6.5(t)

19. Close up the tape job by starting proximally (at the top and progressing distally downwards) overlapping each previous strip, ensuring all gaps ("windows") are covered in order to avoid blisters.
20. Complete the closing-up strips covering the forefoot and distal anchors.

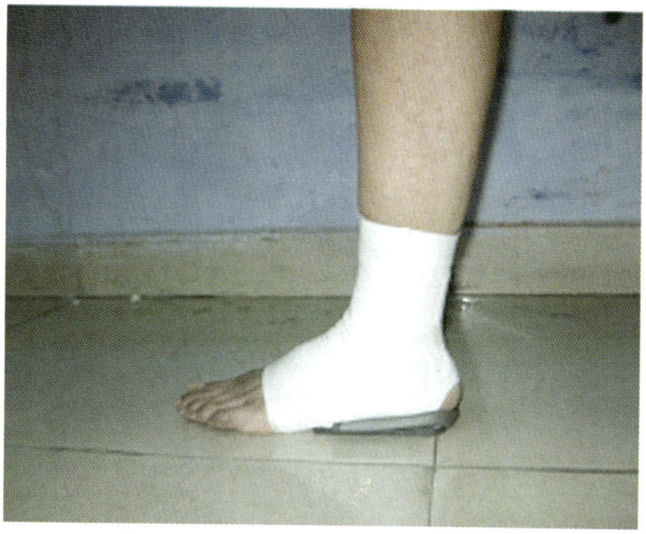

Fig. 6.5(u)

21. Gently at first, test the degree of inversion and plantar flexion restricted by the tape. Add reinforcements if these movements are not adequately limited or if they cause pain.

NOTE: Weight bearing and gradually increasing activity must only be permitted if pain-free both during and after activity.

ANKLE SPRAIN REHABILITATION - ADVANCED SPECIAL ADAPTATION

Sport specific ankle taping variations

During the sub-acute and rehabilitation stage of ankle sprains, the tape job is adapted to the varying needs of the injury. Each tape job must be adjusted for the anatomy of the specific ligament, the degree of injury and the current stage of healing as the athlete gradually returns to sports activity, his sport-specific requirements must also be accommodated.

The following specialized strip adaptations may be used in combination with the previously described strips to adapt to a wide range of situations by the experienced taper.

Specialized strip for sport-specific techniques include:

- **V-lock :** For extra heel stability (useful when number of tape strip must be kept to a minimum i.e. when the athlete must wear the tight boots).
- **Heel locking Figure 8:** Reinforces stability when the level of recovery permits a return to activity.
- **Reverse Figure 8:** Reinforces stability without restricting plantar flexion (useful when plantar flexion is needed for sports participation).

SPECIALIZED STRIPS: V- LOCK (Figs. 6.6(a) to (e))

Purpose

- Reinforce lateral stability.
- Locks the heel.
- Useful when tight fitting footwear is required, as in figure skating and downhill skiing where tape thickness over the malleoli (ankle bones) must be kept to a minimum.

Advantages

- Offers a combination of lateral stability and heel-locking with one single strip.

Disadvantages

- Does not restrict talar tilt as effectively as single ankle lock.

Procedure

1. Place the tape under the heel before pulling up on the anterior end and affixing it to the upper anchor, anteriorly.

Tips: Ensure that the foot is everted (pulled outward) by the pulling of this step.

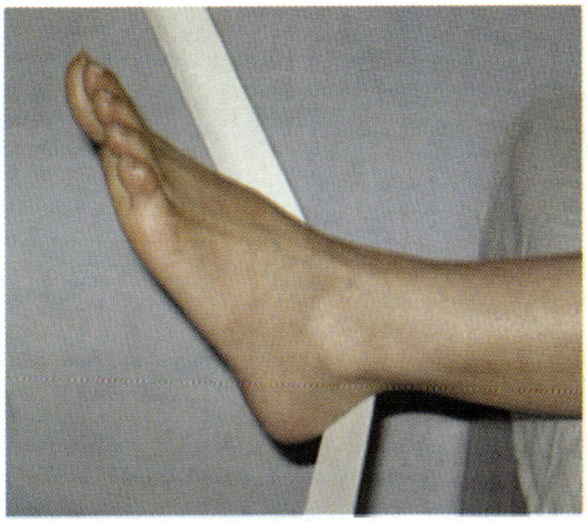

Fig. 6.6(a)

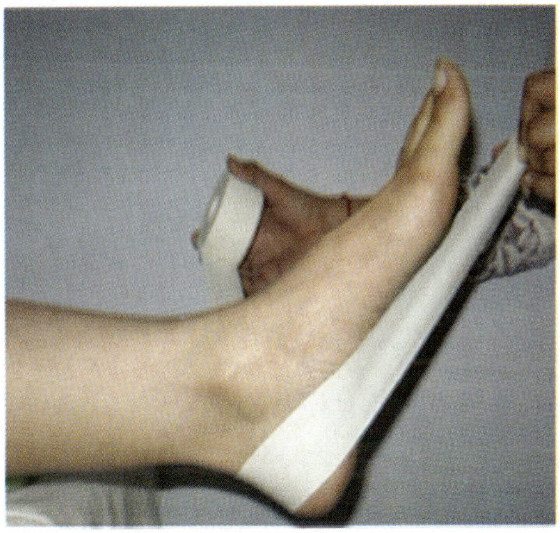

Fig. 6.6(b)

2. Gently wrap the roll of tape behind the heel, crossing low enough on the lateral side to cover the lateral malleolus.

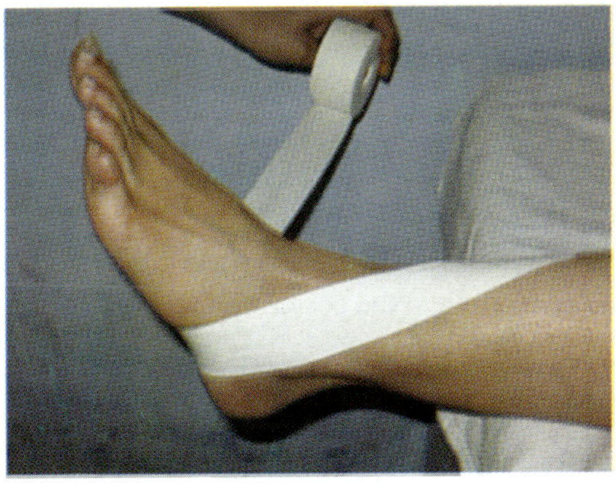

Fig. 6.6(c)

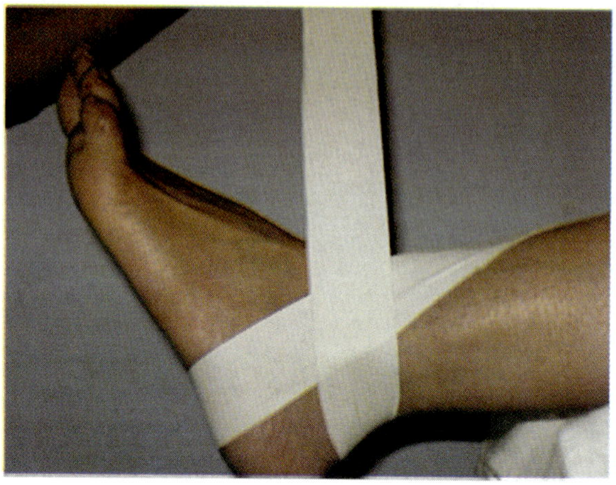

Fig. 6.6(d)

3. Pull the tape snugly across the lateral malleolus to the dorsum of the foot.

Tips: Lateral shearing of the tape and careful attention to the "take-off" direction will help in achieving the best taping "line" without wrinkling the tape.

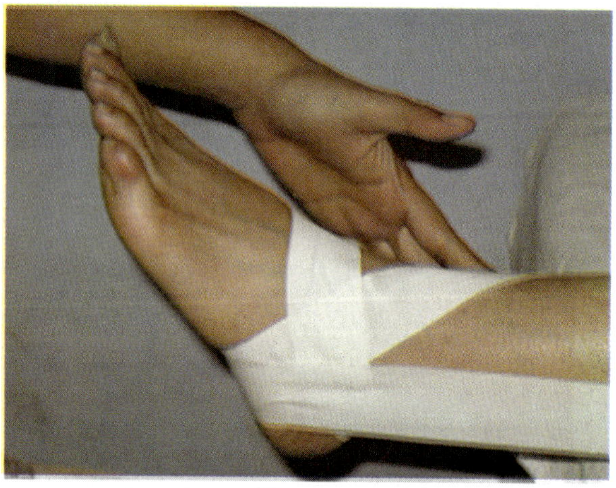

Fig. 6.6(e)

4. Wrap the tape without tension-across the front of the ankle.
5. Pass medially to the plantar (inferior) surface under the arch going in the posterior direction.
6. Now pull up strongly, posterior to lateral malleolus, and adhere the strip to the anchor.

Tips: Repeated application using a practice tape strip will improve technique.

NOTE: This strip can also be applied to the medial side for added stability and heel locking effect. Care must be taken not to allow inversion of the ankle when taping for lateral sprains.

SPECIALIZED SPRIP: Heel-Locking Figure 8

Purpose

- Offers added reinforcement with specific heel stabilization.
- Restricts full plantar.
- Limits lateral mobility.
- Allows almost full dorsiflexion.

Advantage

- Useful in sports requiring more dorsiflexion and where there is less demand for extreme plantar flexion.

Disadvantage

- Restricts plantar flexion.

Procedure

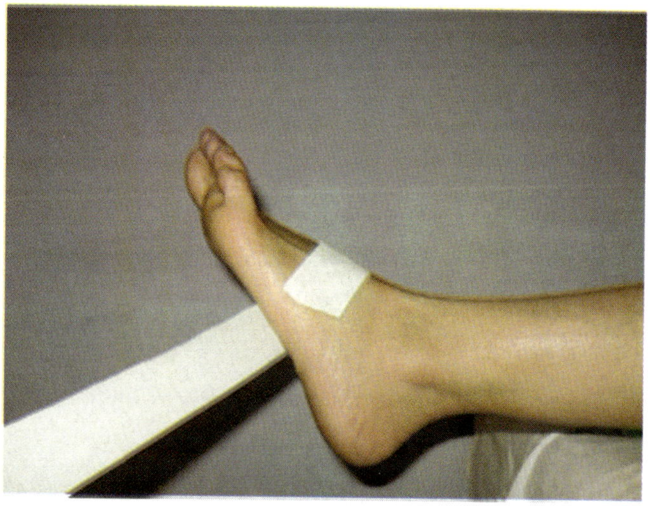

Fig. 6.7(a)

1. Start strip on the dorsum of the foot, from lateral to medial, pass under the instep, and pull up strongly on the lateral side.
2. Carefully cross the tape over the extensor tendons (without wrinkling) and pass horizontally behind the medial to wrap around the Achilles tendon.

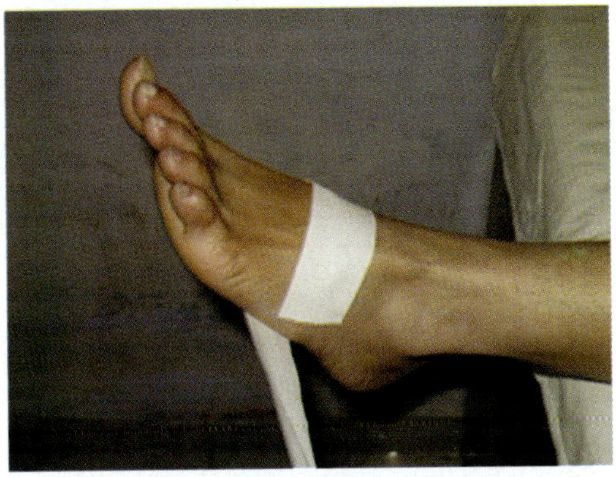

Fig. 6.7(b)

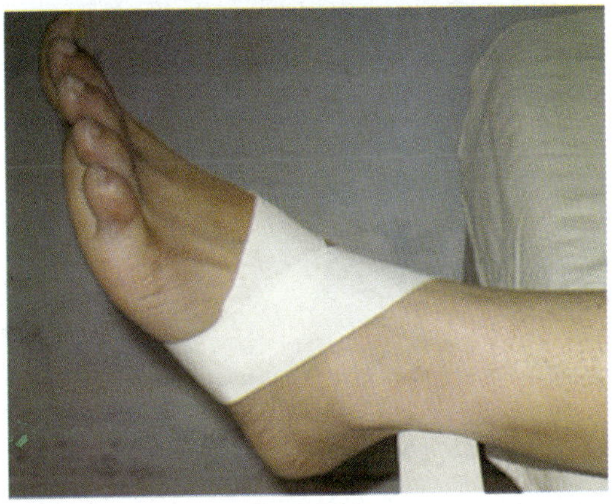

Fig. 6.7(c)

3. Cross the ankle anteriorly, moving down the medial side and under the instep, slightly posterior to the starting point. Angle the tape in the posterior direction under the plantar surface.

Tips: The ankle must be adequately dorsiflexed in order to have the tape pass posteriorly without bending, wrinkling, or causing a pressure ridge.

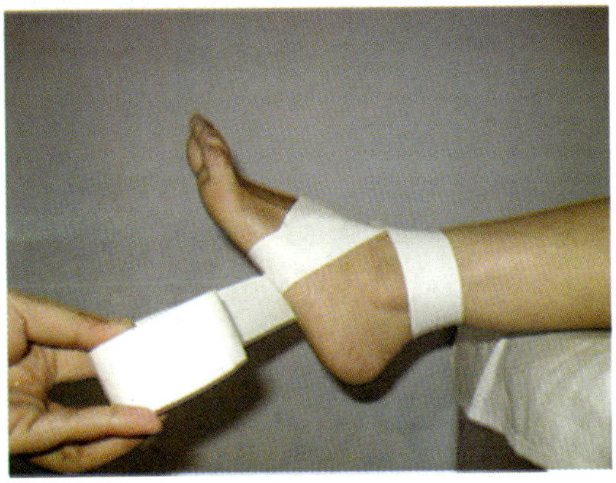

Fig. 6.7(d)

4. Pull the tape up and back with strong tension posterior to the lateral malleolus and pass behind the Achilles tendon.

   Continue carefully around the front of ankle.

Tips: Repeated application using a practice strip will aid in judging the taping angels and will improve proficiency significantly.

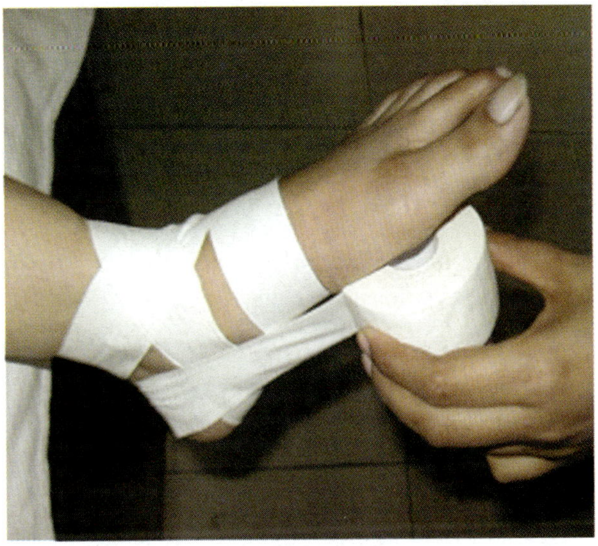

Fig. 6.7(e)

5. Return posteriorly behind the Achilles tendon again, this time crossing the heel from the medial side and with less tension under the instep.

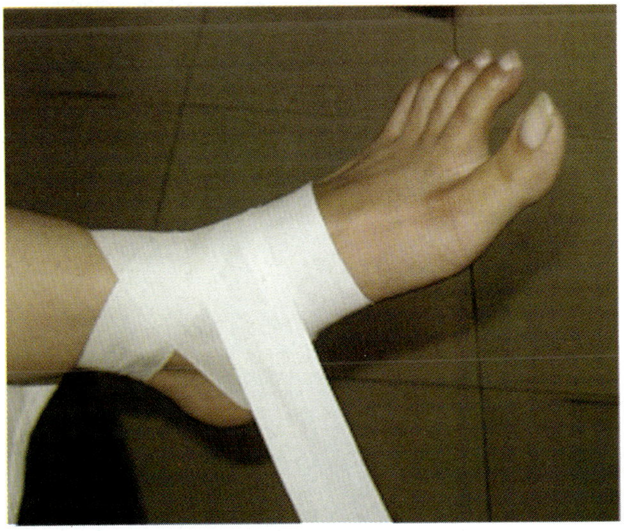

Fig. 6.7(f)

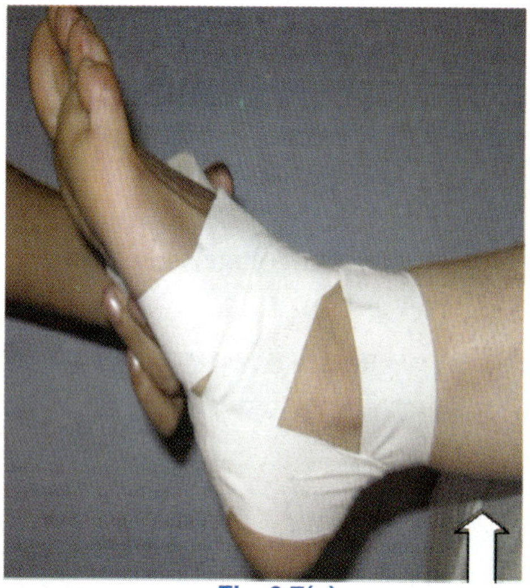

Fig. 6.7(g)

6. Pull up strongly on the lateral side to end by crossing the previous strips anteriorly.

J-LOCK (Figs. 6.8(a) to (c))

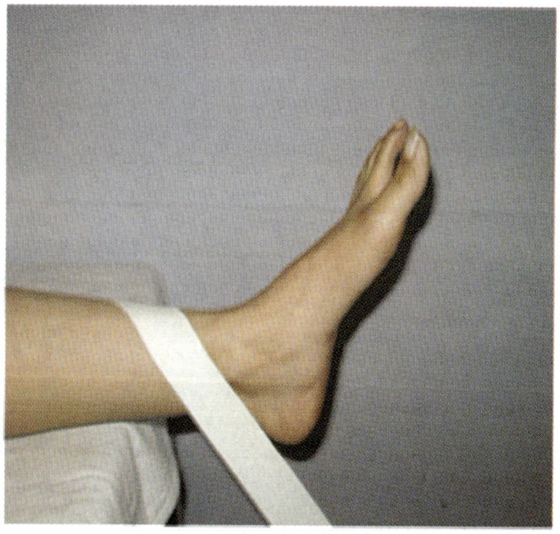

Fig. 6.8(a)

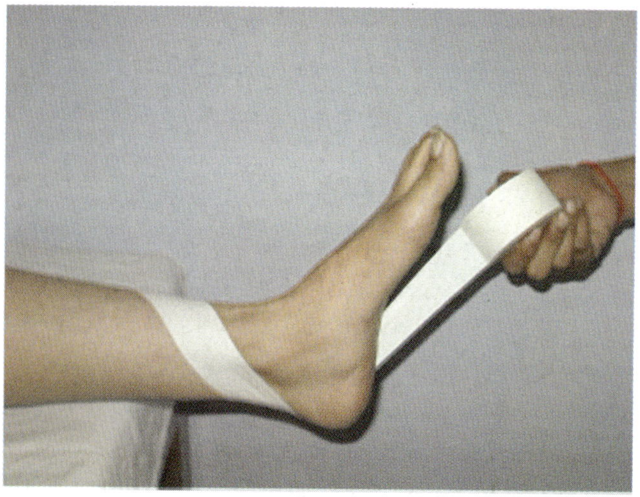

Fig. 6.8(b)

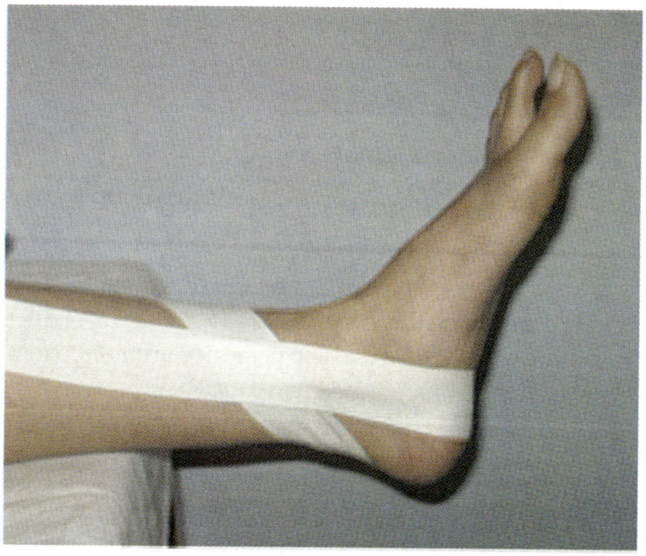

Fig. 6.8(c)

7 LEG TAPING

CALF

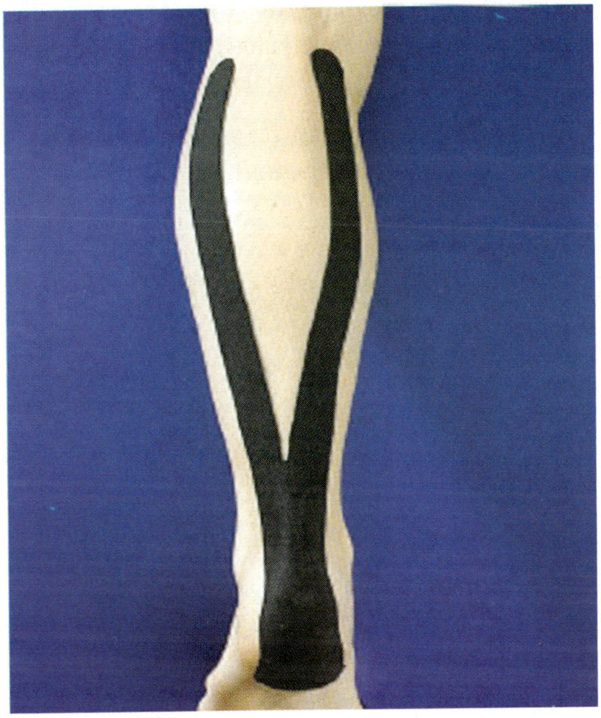

TAPING FOR CALF CONTUSION OR STRAIN

Purpose

- Applies localized specific compression to the bruised or torn tissue (prevents subsequent swelling, bleeding or muscle fiber tearing in the area).
- Supports the triceps surae (calf) muscles with elastic reinforcement assisting plantar flexion.
- Prevents full stretch of musculotendinous unit by restricting dorsiflexion.
- Limits inversion significantly when heel lock is used.
- Allows full plantar flexion and eversion.

Indications for use

- Gastrocnemius or soleus (calf) strain in muscle bulk or musculo-tendinous junction.
- Gastrocnemius or soleus (calf) muscle bulk contusion ("charley-horse").

NOTES:

- The exact site of contusion or strain must be localized.
- Prowrap is not recommended as it significantly lessens the effectiveness of this taping technique.
- Icing of the injured muscles should start immediately.

Flexibility starts as soon as the compression tape is applied by actively conditioning the dorsi-flexors (opposite muscle group).

MATERIALS

Razor.

Skintoughner spray.

(3 inch) elastic adhesive tape.

(1.5 inch) non elastic white tape.

(4 inch) elastic wrap.

(2/3 inch) felt heel lift.

INJURY: CALF STRAIN

TERMINOLOGY

- Gastrocnemius or soleus strain. Also: contusion.
- Achilles tendon complex strain: "pulled" heel cord.
- Degree of severity: 1st to 3rd.
- Torn Achilles tendon 3rd degree strain.

ETIOLOGY

- Sudden forced dorsiflexion during active plantar flexion.
- Explosive plantar flexion against resistance.
- Overstretching.
- External impact to calf (contusion).
- Inadequate warm-up.

SYMPTOMS

- History of sudden sharp pain.
- "Pop" sensation.
- Feeling of being shot in the calf.
- Varying degree of pain at the injury site.
- Local swelling and gradual discolouration.
- Active movement testing.

  No significant pain on non-weight bearing movements

  Calf pain on active plantar flexion if weight bearing

  Calf pain on dorsiflexion if tight calf is being stretched.
- Passive movement testing: Pain on dorsiflexion (1st and 2nd degrees).
- Resistance testing (Neutral position).

  (a) Pain on mild to moderate resistance and weakness of plantar flexion (1st and 2nd degree of severity).

  (b) Inability to plantar flex with little or no pain is inductive of 3rd degree of severity (complex rupture).

TREATMENT

Early

- R.I.C.E.S.
- Taping.
- Heel lift.
- Therapeutic modalities.
- Active contraction of dorsiflexors to induce relaxation and improve flexibility of calf (isometric at first).

Later

- Continued physiotherapy including:
  - Therapeutic modalities.
  - Flexibility.
  - Strengthening.
- Proprioception.
- Rehabilitation program: Non-weight bearing initially, progressive to dynamic pain-free reintegration with taped support for Achilles Tendon Taping.
- Transverse friction massage (only after several weeks when scar tissue is adhering).

SEQUELAE

- Haematoma if massaged too early.
- Inflexibility.
- Weakness.
- Highly prone to re-straining/cramping.

POSITIONING

Lying prone at the end of a low bench with a folded towel placed under the patella (kneecap) and the calf extending over the end of the bench.

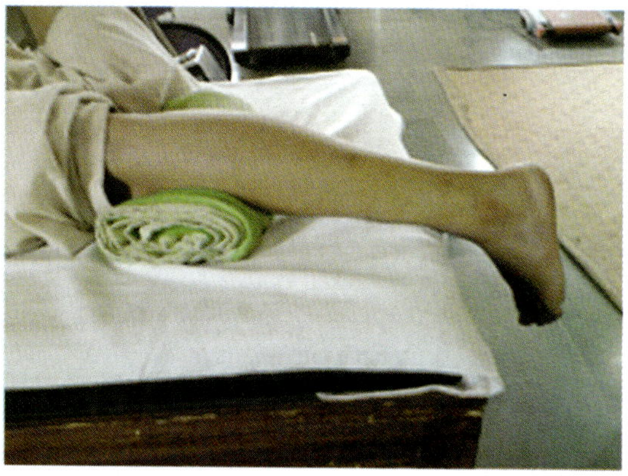

Fig. 7.1(a)

PROCEDURE (Figs. 7.1(a) to (i))

1. Clean shave and dry the area to be taped, checking for cuts, abrasions and sensitive skin.
2. Spray skin toughener or quick dry adhesive spray

circumferentially to the entire calf and let dry completely.

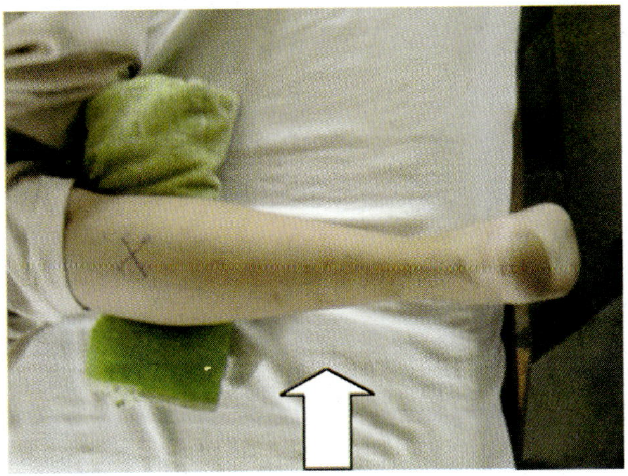

Fig. 7.1(b)

3. Localize the exact site of contusion or muscle strain. Beginning (3 inch) below the lower aspect of injury, using light tension, wrap (3 inch) elastic adhesive tape around the limb. Repeat this strip overlapping the previous one by (2/3 inch) until the entire injured area is covered and surpassed by (3 inch).

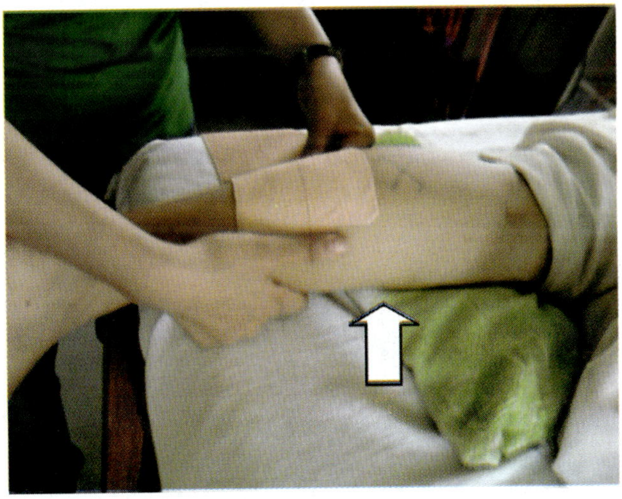

Fig. 7.1(c)

4. Prepare to apply the first strip directly below the center of the site of the injury fold back (4 inch) at the end of a roll of (3 inch) elastic adhesive tape in one band and hold the remainder of the roll in the other.

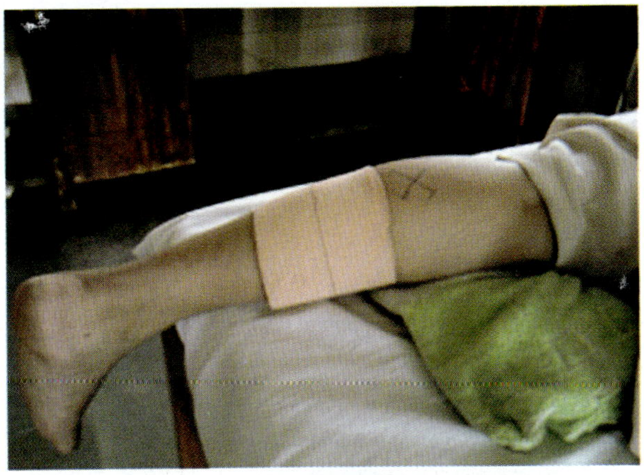

Fig. 7.1(d)

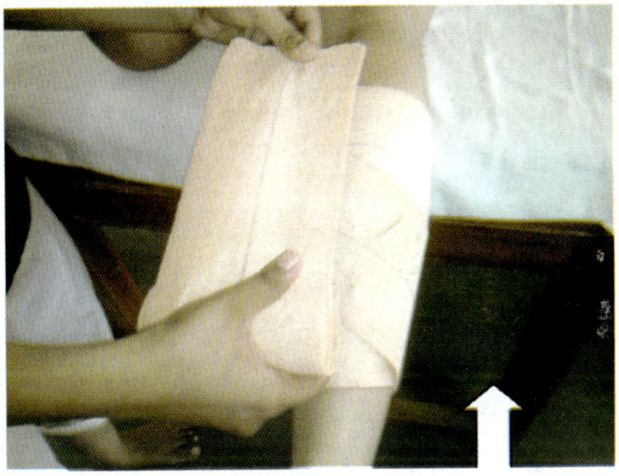

Fig. 7.1(e)

5. Stretch the tape fully and keep it stretched laterally.
6. Apply strong pressure to the limb equally with both hands while maintaining the lateral stretch until the tape reaches the 3/4th of the way around the limb.

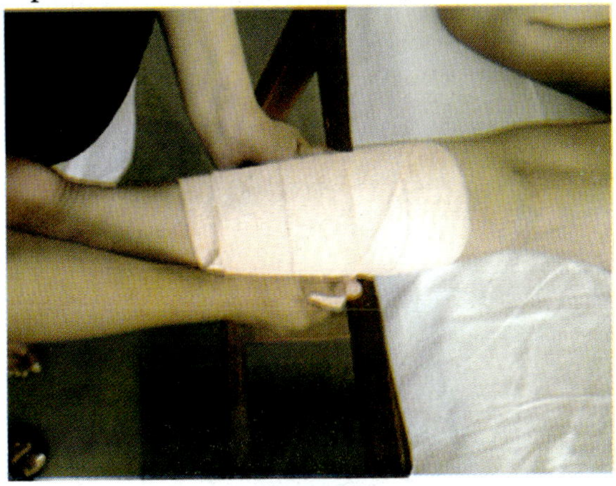

Fig. 7.1(f)

7. Being careful to keep the strip from detaching, release the tension while holding the stretched part against the limb, before adhering the end without any tension at all.

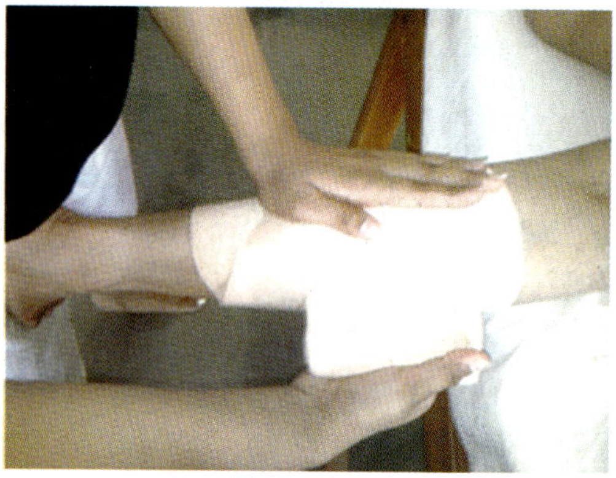

Fig. 7.1(g)

8. Complete encircling the limb with the other end of strip in the same manner, completely overlapping the tape ends at the back.

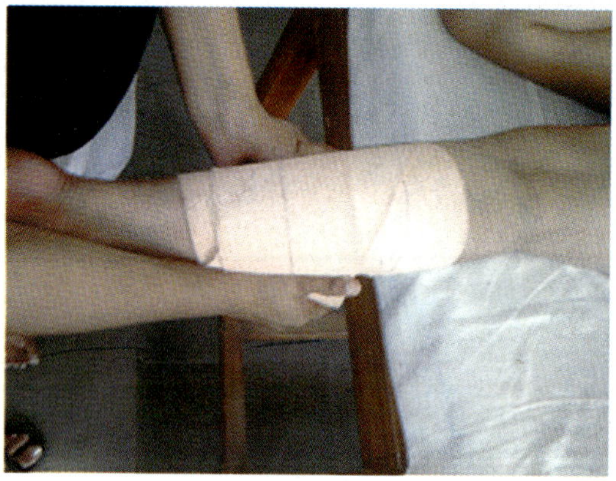

Fig. 7.1(h)

9. Repeat the pressure strip overlapping by half the tapes width above the last strips more proximally, focusing the pressure directly over the injury.

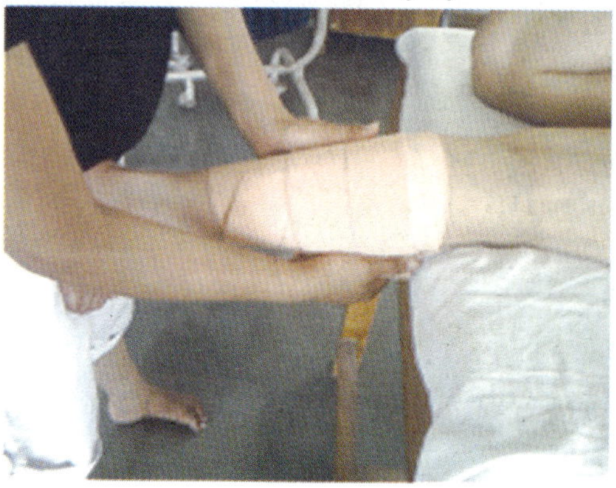

Fig. 7.1(i)

10. Continue repeating the pressure strips more proximally until the base is covered.

TAPING FOR ACHILLES TENDON INJURY

Purpose

- Supports the Achilles tendon with elastic reinforcement assisting plantar flexion.
- Prevents full stretch of the musculo-tendinous unit by restricting full dorsiflexion.
- Limits inversion significantly when heel lock is used.
- Permits full plantar flexion and eversion.

Indications for its use

- Achilles tendon strain.
- Achilles tendinitis.
- Diffuse heel pain (possible bursitis).
- Calf strain: Use in combination with compression taping.
- Calf contusion, use in combination with compression taping.
- Peroneus longus strain or tendinitis, use in combination with peroneus longus support strips.
- Tibialis posterior strain or tendinitis: Use in combination with tibialis posterior support strips.

NOTES:

- Be sure that a thorough assessment has been done. In third degree strain (complete rupture):
  (a) Passive squeezing of the calf in a prone position will not produce plantar flexion of the foot on the injured side (positive Thompson test).
  (b) A palpable gap may be present.
  (c) A passive dorsiflexion will be significantly free on the injured site and does not extreme pain.

If a third degree strain is suspected the athelete must be seen by an orthopedic surgeon as early as possible.

- Evaluate the site of injury; pain may be located at the base of the Achilles tendon, in the belly of the calf muscle, or at the musculo-tendinous junction.
- During taping, neutral alignment can be controlled by the taper whose thigh is used as counter pressure against the athlete great toe.
- Because Achilles taping pulls the foot into plantar flexion, the ankle is rendered less stable and the risk of inversion sprain is increased.
- Once taped, a felt or foam heel-lift in the athlete's shoe will shorten and help support the Achilles tendon by improving its mechanical advantage.

TERMINOLOGY

- Achilles tendon inflammation (irritation).
- Chronic heel cord strain.

ETIOLOGY

- Structural strain from repeated quick push-offs as in repetitive running.
- Sudden change in training; increased distance, speed or intensity; change of terrain (example: hills vs. level ground).
- New footwear—Inadequate heel support.
- Inadequate warm-up and stretchings.
- Subsequent to a gastrocnemius (calf) strain.

SYMPTOMS

- Tenderness plus swelling around tendon.
- Localized pain (usually mid-tendon) spreads as condition progresses.
- Acute posterior heel pain on weight bearing plantar flexion (particularly after resting).
- Active motion testing: Possible pain on plantar flexion.
- Passive movement testing (neutral position): Possible weakness marked pain on moderate resistance.

TREATMENT

- Physiotherapy including:
  - Ice.
  - Therapeutic modalities.
  - Transverse friction massage.
- Achilles tendon taping.
- Heel lift.
- Modified training program.
- Total rehabilitation program with emphasis on full flexibility, eccentric strengthening through range of motion and dynamic proprioception.
- Progressive reintegration to regular sports activity with taped support as above.

SEQUELAE

- Persistent pain.
- Scarring/thickening of tendon.
- Inflexibility.
- Weakness of calf.
- Imbalance of ankle musculature flexibility and/or strength.
- Bursitis.
- Calcification of tendon or bursa.

POSITIONING

Lying prone with foot protruding over the edge of the table.

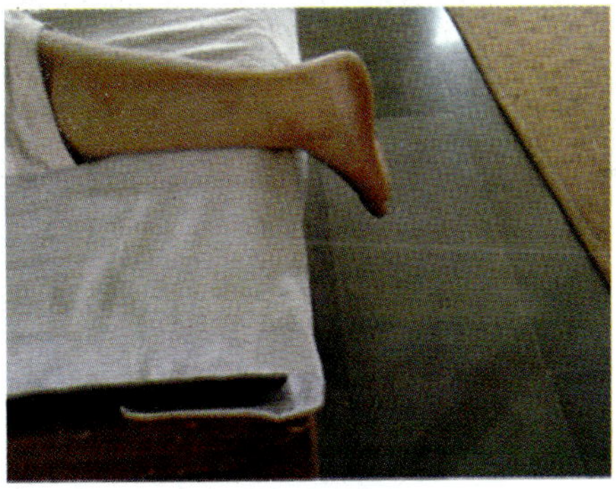

Fig. 7.2(a)

PROCEDURE (Figs. 7.2(a) to (m))

1. Clean, shave and dry the area, checking for skin irritations, cuts or abrasions.
2. Spray with skin toughener or quick dry adhesive.
3. Apply prowrap without tension around ankle upto lower 1/3 of calf.

NOTE: Heel and lace pads should be used when taping is to enable athlete to resume playing.

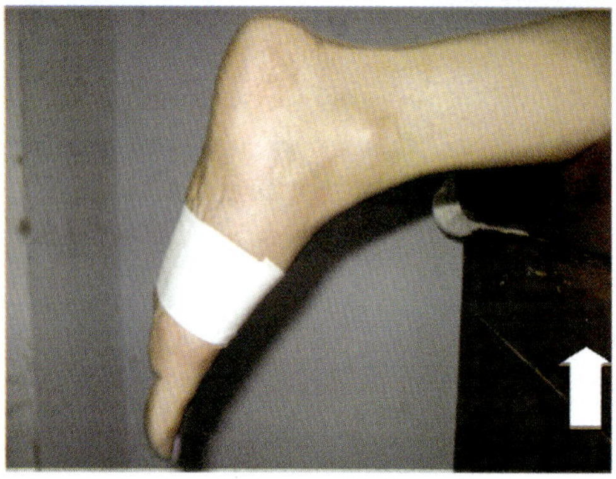

Fig. 7.2(b)

4. Apply two circumferential anchors of (1.5 inch) white tape at the level of heads of metatarsals.

Tip: Be sure to allow for some splaying of the metatarsals.

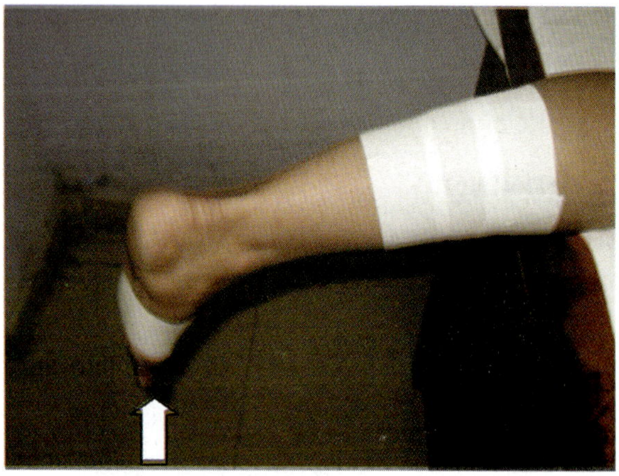

Fig. 7.2(c)

5. Have the athlete turn to lie prone to facilitate the rest of the taping technique. Using only slight tension, apply two circumferential anchors of (2 inch) elastic adhesive tape at mid-belly of calf muscle.

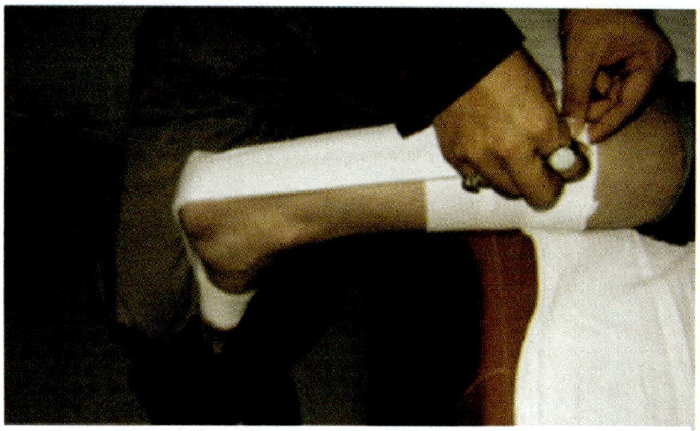

Fig. 7.2(d)

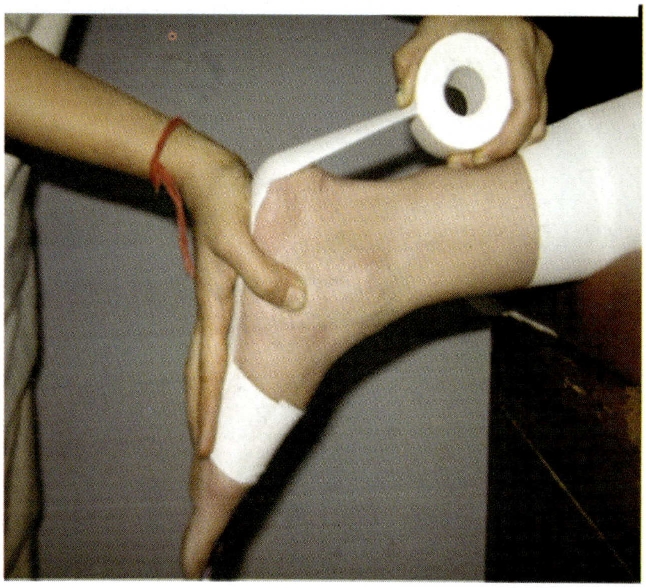

Fig. 7.2(e)

6. Apply the first vertical strip using (3 inch) adhesive elastic tape.
   (a) Fix it firmly, **without tension**, to the plantar surface of foot.
   (b) Pull upwards from center of the back of the calcaneus (heel), **with strong tension** with lower edge of the calf anchor.

Tip: Allow the ankle to plantar flex.

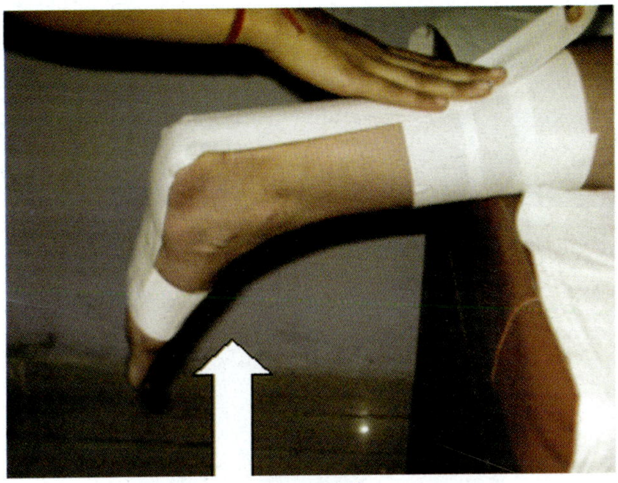

Fig. 7.2(f)

(c) Support this strip without loosening its tension and carefully apply the last 5 cm (2 inch) of tape without virtually any tension, before cutting the tape from the roll.

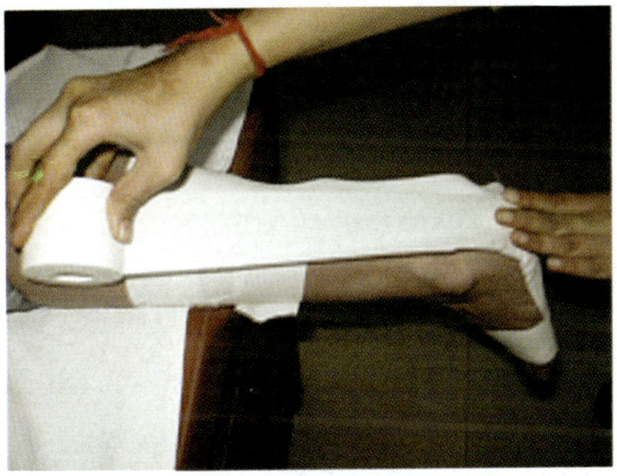

Fig. 7.2(g)

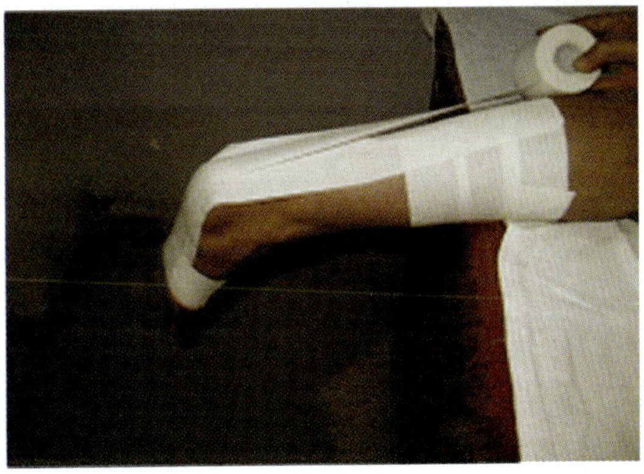

Fig. 7.2(h)

7. Passing just medially to the centre of back of heel, pulling up firmly to control the lateral tilt of the calcaneus.

Tip: Maintain strong tension while adhering the upper end of this strip to the calf anchors cutting the tape

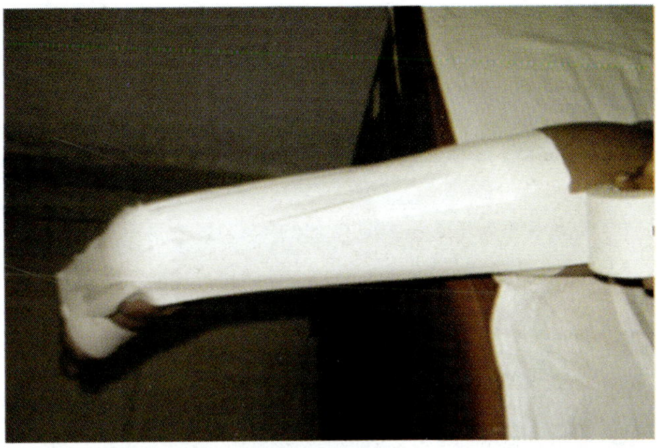

Fig. 7.2(i)

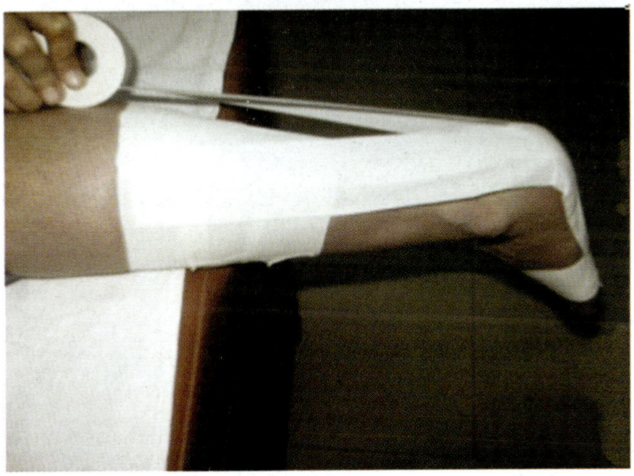

Fig. 7.2(j)

8. Passing just lateral to centre of back of heel, controlling the lateral tilt and forming a "v" over the Achilles tendon posteriorly before reanchoring strips at both ends.

NOTE: Special reinforcement strips should be added after this strip before going on to step 9.

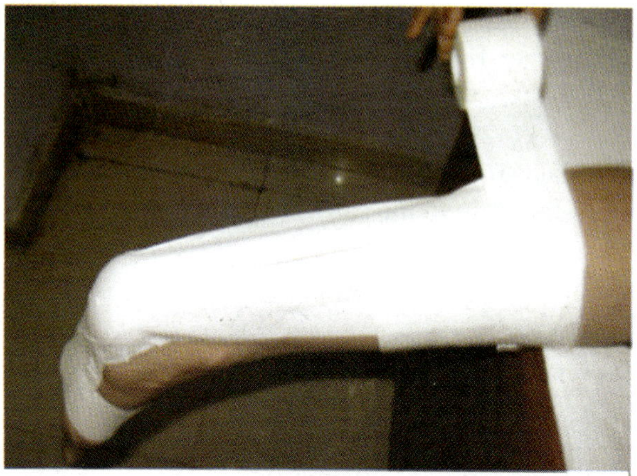

Fig. 7.2(k)

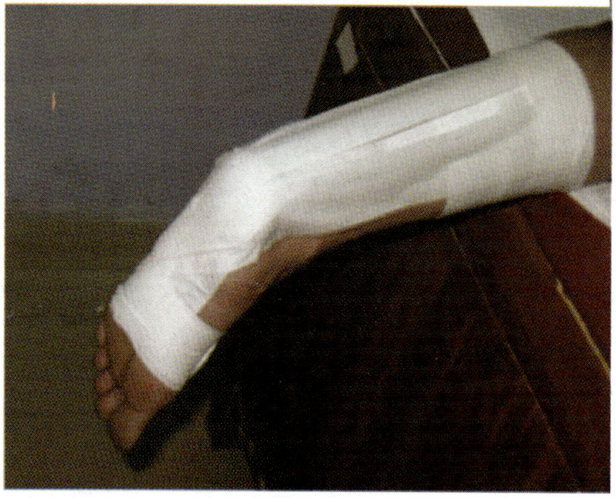

Fig. 7.2(l)

9. Close up calf portion of the tape job with circumferential strips of elastic adhesive tape.
10. Reposition the athlete in a supine (lying face up) position to facilitate the next steps.
11. Close up foot portion of the tape job with circumferential strips of white tape, overlapping each previous strip.
12. A lateral ankle lock is applied to offer stability.
13. Reanchor these locks.

NOTE: A medial lock can also be applied to reinforce stability in particularly vulnerable ankles.

14. Close up the entire tape job, covering any open areas.

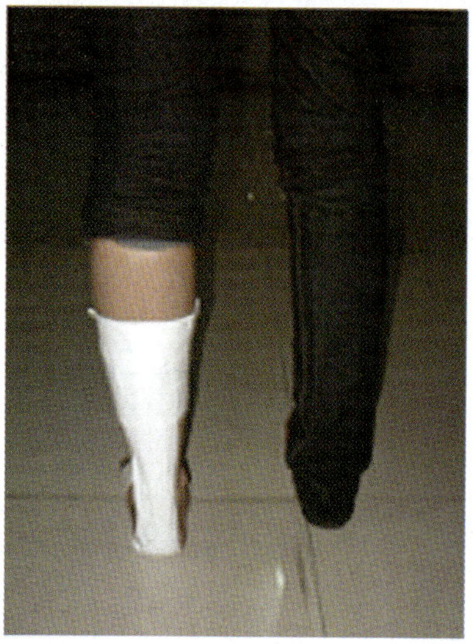

Fig. 7.2(m)

15. Test limit of taping restriction to ensure adequate pain free support.
    (a) Dorsiflexion must be limited by at least 30 degree.
    (b) There should be no pain on passive dorsiflexion.
16. For acute and sub acute stages cut a felt heel lift, beveled at the anterior (front) edge, and place it under the heel to raise it thereby reducing tension on the tendon.

Tip: It is best to add heel lifts to both feet for a balanced gait.

8 Knee and Thigh Taping

KNEE AND THIGH

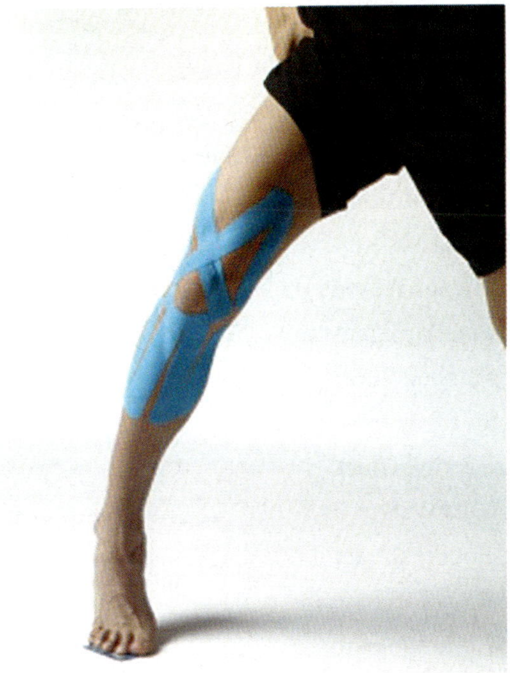

Fig. 8.1

The knee is a hinged weight bearing joint dependent on several structures for stability.

- **Medial and lateral collateral ligaments** prevent lateral (sideways) movement.
- **Anterior and posterior cruciate ligaments** located centrally, prevent anterior (forward) and posterior (backward) displacement during movement.
- **Two wedge shaped menisci (cartilages)** from mechanical spacers cushion forces, guide movements and add to total stability.

The **patella (knee cap)**, while improving the biomechanical efficiency of the quadriceps, is often the source of incapacity knee pain.

The knee is frequently injured–especially in contact sports–due to several factors:

- Heavy weight bearing demands on the knee in sports activities.
- A relatively weaker medial collateral ligament with its attachments to the medial meniscus.
- Vulnerability of the anterior cruciate ligament.

Correct taping and treatment for knee sprains permits the athlete to continue sports participation with minimal risk of sustaining further injury. Taped support gives stability to the injured structure, enhances end-range proprioceptive feedback, and promotes healing through dynamic function.

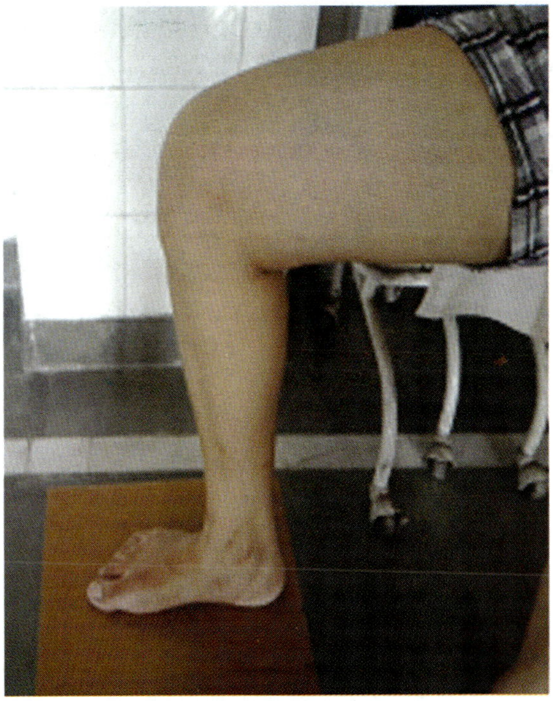

Fig. 8.2(a): Medial side, right knee

X=Crossed Taping

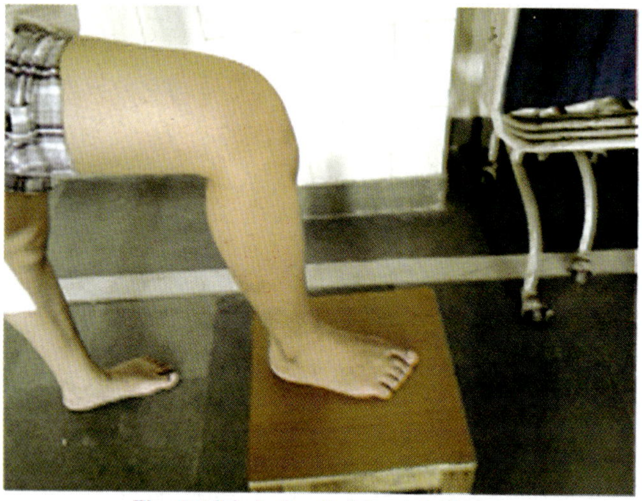

Fig. 8.2(b): Lateral side, right knee

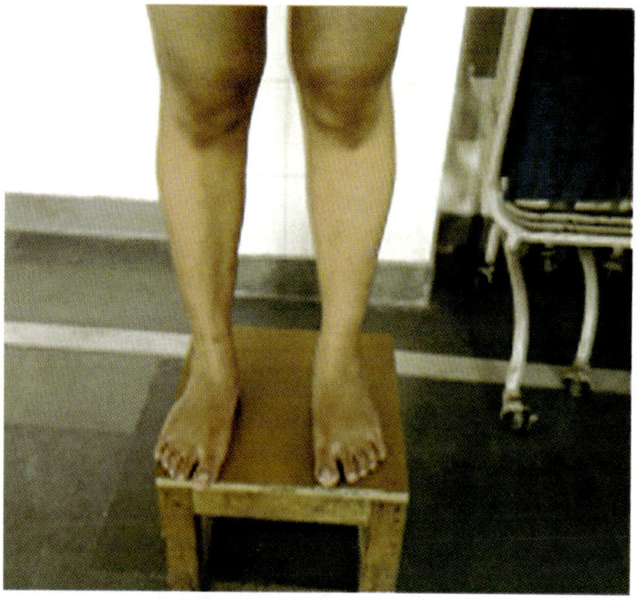

Fig. 8.2(c): Anterior view of knee

MUSCLES

1. Quadriceps: Rectus femoris
2. Quadriceps: Vastus medialis
3. Quadriceps: Vastus lateralis
4. Gastrocnemius
5. Semimembranosis
6. Adductor magnus

BONES

7. Patella
8. Margin of condyle of femur
9. Tuberosity of tibia
10. Margin of condyle of tibia
11. Head of fibula

TENDONS

12. Biceps femoris
13. Patellar ligament
14. Semitendinosis

FASCIA

15. Illiotibial tract

HOLLOWS

16. Popliteal tract

NERVES

17. Common peroneal

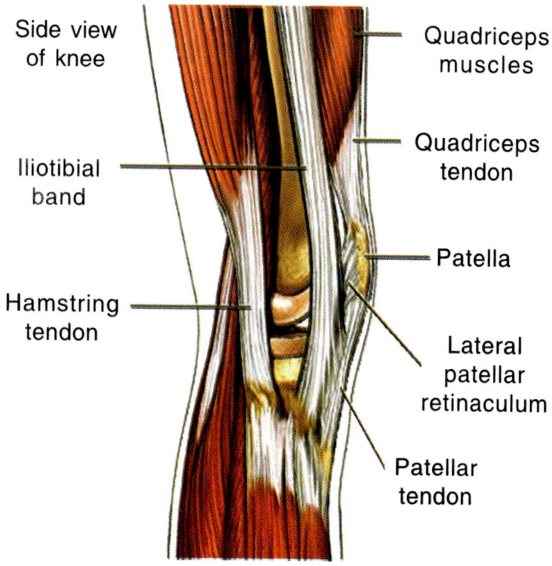

Behind the knee on the lateral side the rounded tendon, of biceps can be felt easily, with the broad strap–like iliotibial tract in front of it, with a furrow between them. On the medial side two tendons can be felt–the narrow rounded semitendinosus just behind the border semimembranosus. At the front of patellar ligament keep the patella at a constant distance from the tibia tuberosity, while at the adjutant's margin of the femoral and tibia and condyle can be palpated.

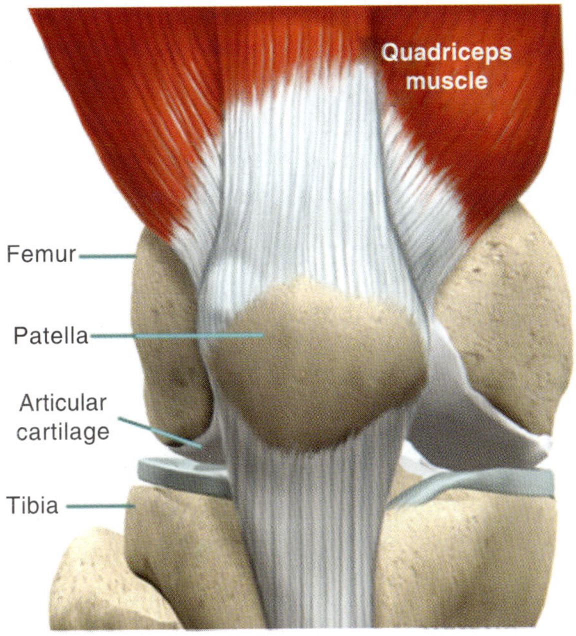

TAPING FOR MEDIAL COLLATERAL LIGAMENT (MCL) KNEE SPRAIN

Purpose

- Supports the medial collateral (MCL) by tightening the medial aspect of the joint line.
- Prevents the last 15 degree of knee extension and external rotation of tibia under the femur.
- Allows almost full flexion and functional extension of the knee.

Indications for use

- Medial collateral ligament (MCL) sprains: 1st and 2nd degree.
- Post immobilization of 3rd degree MCL sprain.
- For medial meniscus injuries: Emphasize spiral strips which cause internal rotation of the tibia.

MATERIALS

- Razor.
- Skin toughener spray.
- Prowrap.
- (3 inch) and (4 inch) elastic adhesive tape.
- (2 inch) and (1.5 inch) non-elastic white tape.
- (6 inch) elastic wrap.
- Skin lubricant.

NOTES:
To determine the degree of injury, be certain that a competent sports physiotherapist examines the athlete.

a. Medial stability should be tested at 30 degree of knee flexion as well as at 0 degree.
b. If the knee is also unstable at 0 degree of extension, a serious injury is suspected.
c. X-rays should be taken to rule out an avulsion fracture.
   - Always assess which knee and which side of that knee was injured (the athlete may have sustained spraining on the medial aspect of the same knee and bruising on the lateral aspect).
   - During exercise, increased blood circulation causes swelling of thigh muscles. Ensure that circumferential strips are affixed with only light tension, avoiding constriction of thigh and calf muscles.

INJURY: KNEE SPRAIN MEDIAL COLLATERAL LIGAMENT (MCL)

TEMINOLOGY

- Medial collateral ligament sprain: 1st-3rd degree of severity.
- Internal collateral ligament sprain: 1st-3rd degree of severity.
- Pulled knee.

ETIOLOGY

- Excessive inward pressure forcing the knee medially into valgus (inwardly bent "knock-kneed" position).
- Sudden impact forcing body laterally on a fixed foot.
- Often associated with other injured structures (medial meniscus, anterior cruciate Medial Collateral Ligament (MCL) : "the unhappy triad".

SYMPTOMS

- Local pain and tenderness on the medial side (inside) of the knee.
- Swelling, possible bruising.
- Active movement testing: Medial pain on end-range extension.
- Resistance testing (neutral position): No pain moderate resistance.
- Stress testing:
  a. 1st and 2nd degree sprain: Medial pain with or without instability when tested at 30 degree knee flexion.
  b. 3rd degree of severity: Complete ligament rupture ("open up"); at 30 degree can be less pain than with 2nd degree.
  c. **Instability at 0 degree** extension is indicative of a severe injury with posterior capsule involvement.

TREATMENT

Early

- R.I.C.E.S.
- Taping **MCL** sprain.
- Therapeutic modalities.

> **NOTE:** Surgery may be indicated for 3rd degree of severity.

Later

Continued physiotherapy including:

- Therapeutic modalities.
- Transverse friction massage.
- Mobilizations if stiff following immobilization.
- Flexibility exercises for quadriceps, hamstrings and gastrocnemeius.
- Strengthening exercises (isometric at first) for quadriceps and hamstrings.
- Gradual reintegration program with pain free taped support for MCL.
- Sprain.
- Total rehabilitation program for range of motion, flexibility, strength and proprioception.
- Bracing may be recommended for return to activity or for continued athletic performance if chronically unstable.

SEQUELAE

- Medial (valgus) laxity.
- Chronic instability.
- Weakness of quadriceps.
- Degeneration of medial meniscus.
- Osteoarthritis changes.

POSITIONING (Figs. 8.3(a) to (h))

Standing on a stool or a chair with a roll of tape under the heel (injured side) with the knee bent slightly. The foot is turned inwards to medially rotate the tibia under the femur. (This takes the tension off the medial collateral ligament). 80% of body weight should be supported by the uninjured side.

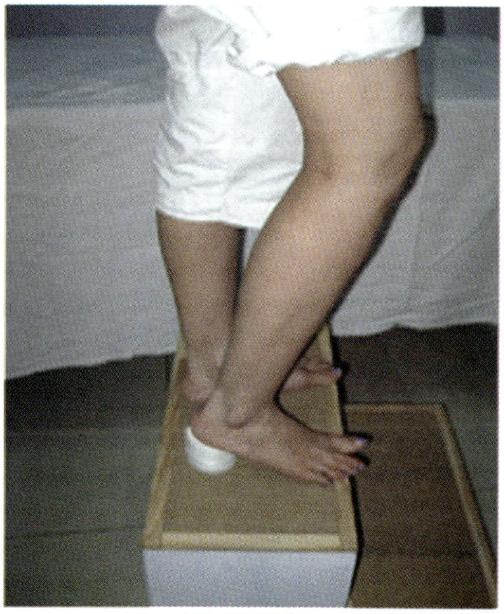

Fig. 8.3(a)

PROCEDURE

1. Clean, shave and dry the area to be taped, checking for cuts, abrasions or sensitive areas.
2. Place lubricated pads over the hamstring tendons.
3. Spray mid-thigh and mid-calf circumferentially with skin toughener or quick dry adhesive.

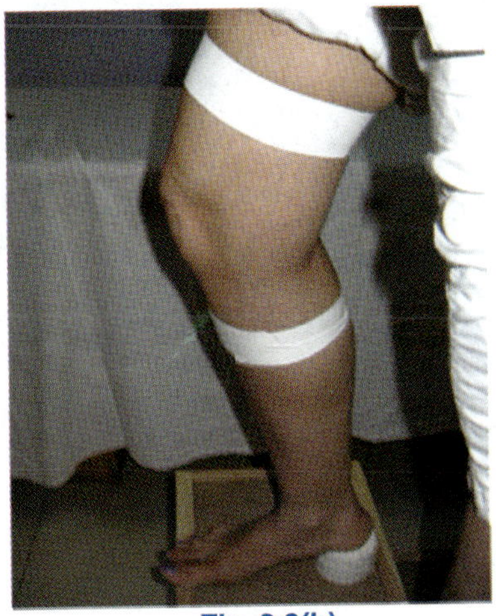

Fig. 8.3(b)

4. Apply 2 circumferential anchors of (4 inch) elastic adhesive tape one using only slight tension, to the mid-calf regions covering the skin well beyond the edge of the prowrap and the 2nd strip on the lower thigh or just above the knee joint.

NOTE: Re-check the athlete's position.

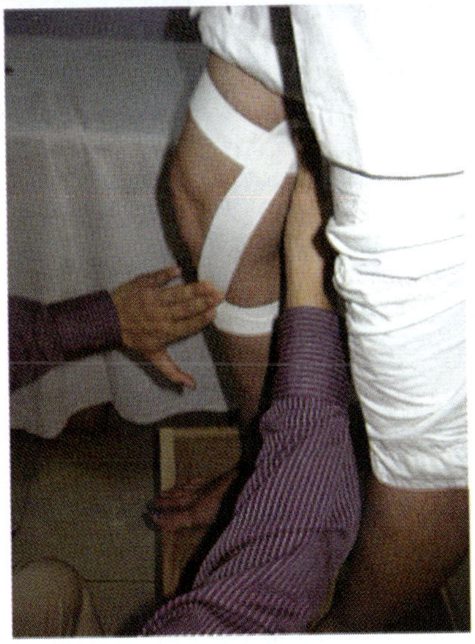

Fig. 8.3(c)

5. Place the strip of (3 inch) elastic adhesive tape starting from the posterior-medial aspect of distal anchors, spiralling around the lateral side of tibia anteriorly. Cross medially below the patella with moderate tension, and pull proximally with strong tension over the medial joint line to the proximal anchor.

NOTE: This strip helps to medially rotate the tibia as well as approximate the medial joint.

Tips: The last 7.5 cm (3 inch) of the strip must be applied directly to the anchor strip, and must not be applied under tension. (The tape end will peel back if the tension has not been released).

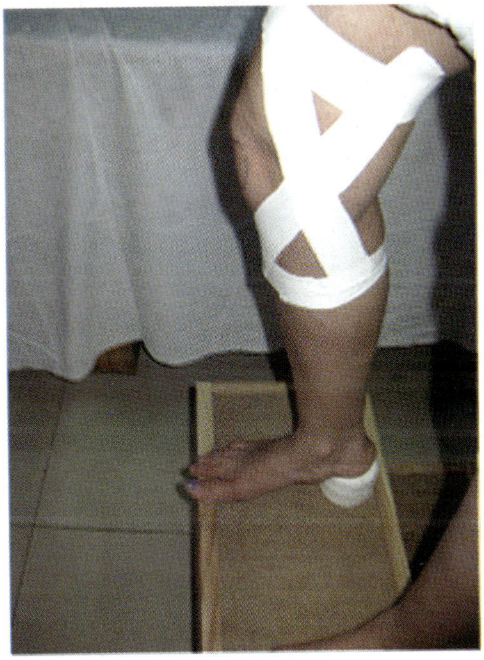

Fig. 8.3(d)

6. Place the second strip of (3 inch) elastic adhesive tape also starting from the posterior-medial aspect of the distal anchor, this time heading anteriorly on the medial side. Pull proximally with a strong tension over the medial joint line to proximal anchor anteriorly, releasing the tension only when adhering the end of the strip.

NOTE: These two strips form a X on the medial joint line, over the site of the medial collateral ligament.

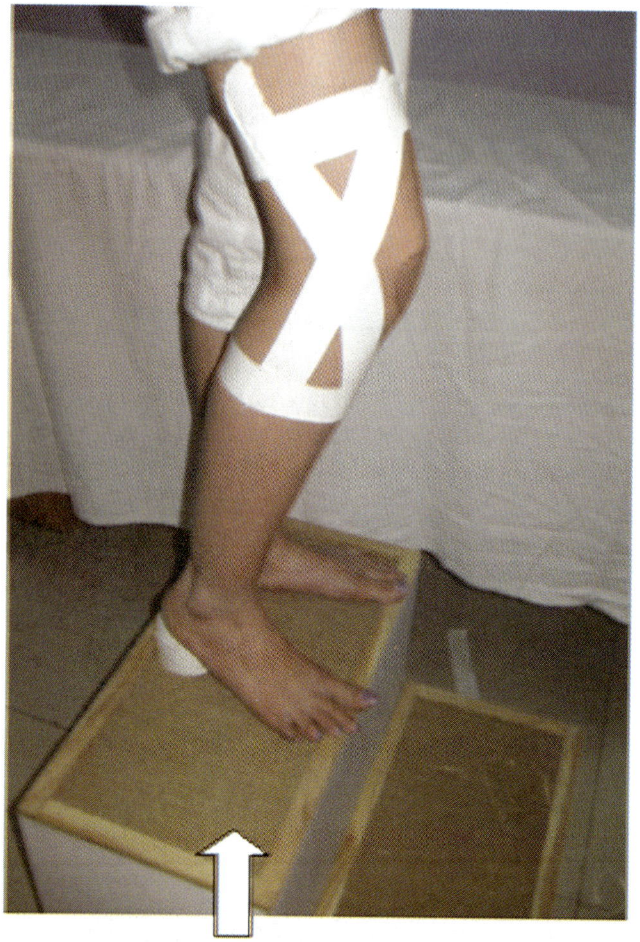

Fig. 8.3(e)

7. Begin a lateral X with a (3 inch) elastic adhesive tape from the posterior-medial aspect of the lower leg, winding behind the tibia (reinforcing internal rotation of the tibia) with some tension upwards on the lateral aspect of the knee above the patella to the proximal anchor anteriorly.
8. Place the next strip of (3 inch) elastic adhesive tape from the anterio lateral aspect of the distal anchor, pulling proximally with some tension over the lateral joint line, to the proximal anchor.

NOTE: These two strips form a X directly on the lateral joint line, with less tension. The ends interlock with the medial X over the anchors, reinforcing stability.

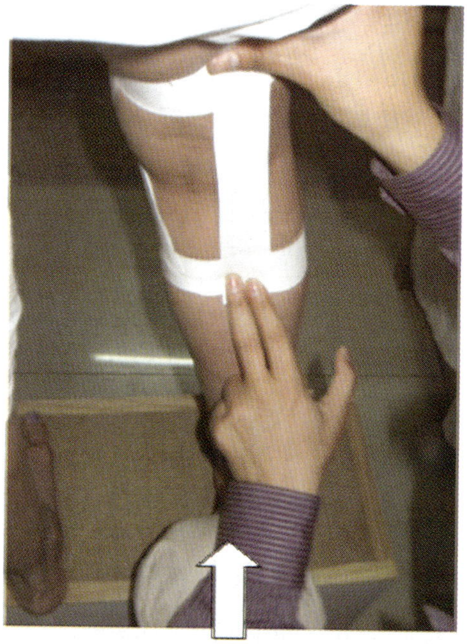

Fig. 8.3(f)

9. With the knee still fixed, apply a vertical strip of (3 inch) elastic adhesive tape from the center of the posterior of the distal anchor to the center of the proximal anchor to prevent hyperextension.

NOTE: Flex the knee at least 30 degree and use strong tension when applying this strip.

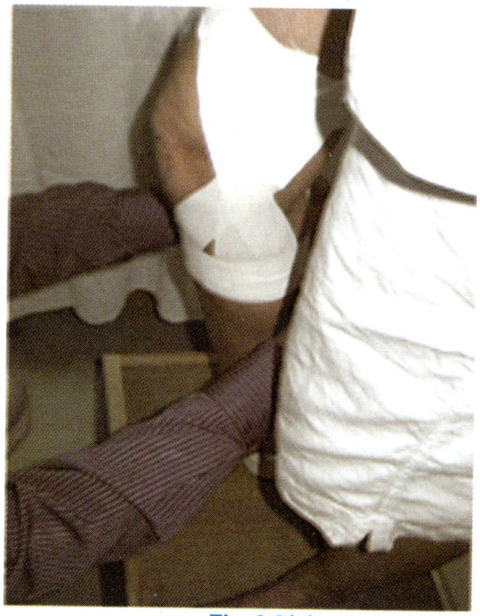

Fig. 8.3(g)

10. Re-anchor the tape with proximal and distal anchors.

NOTE: The athlete will need to hold onto the taper's shoulder or use a nearby wall for stability at this stage.

NOTE: The knee must remain relaxed, while the athlete's weight is borne mainly on the uninjured leg.

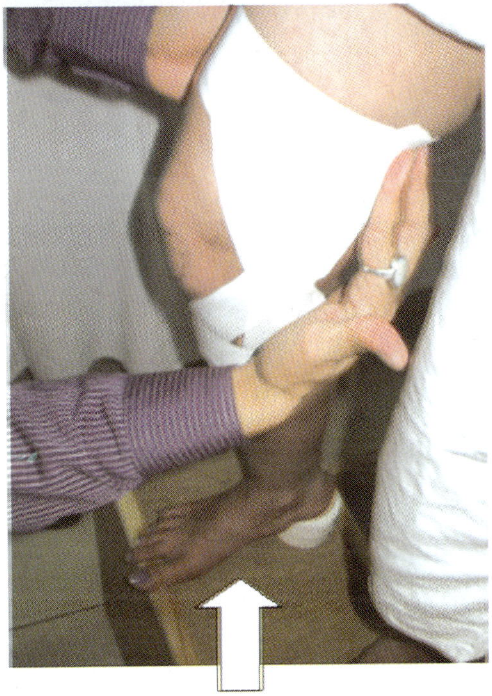

Fig. 8.3(h)

11. Using light tension, re-anchor the tape job with 2 circumferential strips of (4 inch) elastic adhesive tape over the mid thigh anchor and 2 strips over the mid-calf anchor.
12. Cover the end of the elastic tape with two short strips of white tape to keep the elastic tape securely in place.
13. Test the degree of restriction:
    a. Extension must be limited by 10 degree.
    b. There must be no medial laxity.
    c. There must be no pain on medial stress testing inward bending of the knee, external rotation of the tibia under the femur and extension.

TAPING FOR LATERAL COLLATERAL LIGAMENT (LCL) SPRAINS OF THE KNEE

Purpose

- Supports the lateral collateral ligament (LCL) by tightening the lateral aspect of the joint line.
- Prevents the last 15 degree of knee extension and restricts end range flexion slightly.
- Allows functional flexion and extension of the knee.

Indications for use

- Lateral collateral ligament sprains: 1st and 2nd degree.
- Post immobilization of 3rd degree LCL sprains.
- Posterior cruciate ligament sprains.
- Can be combined effectively with taping MCL and/or ACL above for multiple ligament knee injuries.
- Posterior-lateral capsular injuries (combined with ACL taping).

NOTES:

To determine degree of injury, be certain that a competent sports physiotherapist examines the athlete:

(a) Lateral stability should be tested at 30 degree knee flexion and at 0 degree.

(b) If the knee is also unstable medially at 0 degree extension, a serious injury is suspected.

(c) X-rays should be taken.

- Be certain to check both medial and lateral sides of both knees for damage resulting from lateral impact.
- Watch for peroneal nerve damage, weakness of eversion (outward pushing) of foot and decreased sensation-lateral side of injured leg.
- Ensure that the anchor tightness does not compromise circulation.

MATERIALS

- Razor.
- Skin toughener spray.
- Pro wrap.
- Lubricant.
- Heel and lace pads.
- 4 inch elastic adhesive tape.
- 3 inch elastic adhesive tape.
- 2 inch non-elastic white tape.
- 6 inch elastic wrap.

TERMINOLOGY

- Lateral collateral ligament sprain.
- External collateral ligament sprain.
- Fibular collateral ligament sprain.
- Torsicn injury.

ETIOLOGY

- Excessive outward pressure forcing the knee laterally into varus (outward bent or "bow-legged" position).
- Sudden impact forcing body medially on fixed lower leg.
- Direct blow to side of knee.
- Isolated tears are uncommon.

SYMPTOMS

- Pain, tenderness on lateral side (outside) of the knee.
- Swelling, possible bruising.
- Active movement testing: Lateral pain on end-range extension.
- Passive movement testing: Lateral pain on end range extension.
- Resistance testing (neutral position); no pain on moderate resistance.
- Stress testing at 10 degree and 30 degree knee flexion:
  a. 1st and 2nd degree sprains pain or without instability.
  b. 3rd degree of severity: Complete ligament rupture ("open up"); can be less pain than with 2nd degree sprain.
  c. Instability at 0 degree extension is indicative of a severe injury with posterior capsule involvement.

TREATMENT

Early

- R.I.C.E.S.
- Therapeutic modalities.

NOTE: Surgery may be indicated for 3rd degree of severity.

- Taping for LCL sprain.

Later

Continued physiotherapy including:

- Therapeutic modalities.
- Transverse friction massage.
- Mobilizations if stiff post immobilization hamstrings.
- Flexibility exercises for quadriceps, hamstrings, and gastrocnemeius.
- Strengthening of quadriceps, hamstrings and gastrocnemius.
- Strengthening of quadriceps (isometric first).
- Gradual reintegration program with pain free taped support: **ACL SPRAIN TAPING.**
- Total rehabilitation program for range of motion, flexibility, strength and proprioception.
- Bracing may be recommended for return to activity or for continued athletics if chronically unstable.

SEQUELAE

- Lateral (varus) laxity.
- Rotational instability.

- Predisposition to lateral meniscal tears.
- Weakness of quadriceps.
- Instability to "cut" when running.
- Possible peroneal nerve damage.
- Degenerative arthritic changes.

POSITIONING

Standing on a stool or a chair with a roll of tape under the heel (injured side) with the knee bent slightly. The foot is turned outwards to laterally rotate the tibia under femur. (This takes the tension of the lateral collateral ligament). 80% of body weight should be supported by the uninjured side.

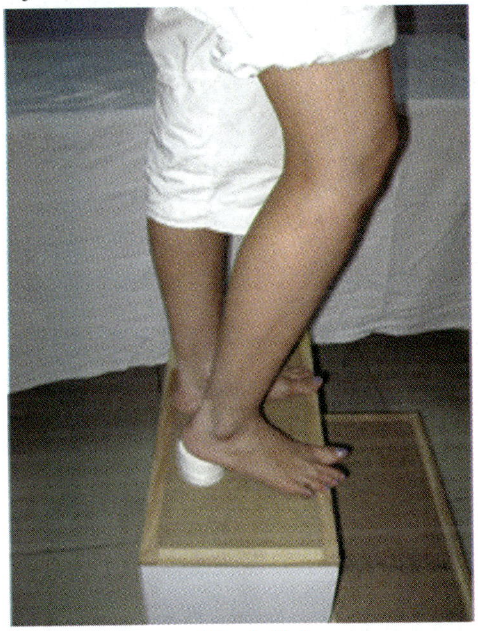

Fig. 8.4(a)

PROCEDURE (Figs. 8.4(a) to (k))

1. Clean shave and dry skin to be taped checking for cuts, abrasions and sensitive areas.
2. Apply skin toughener, skin lubricant pads, prowrap and anchors.

Tips: Apply lubricant and padding on both hamstring tendons to protect tender skin from irritation, blisters and tape cuts.

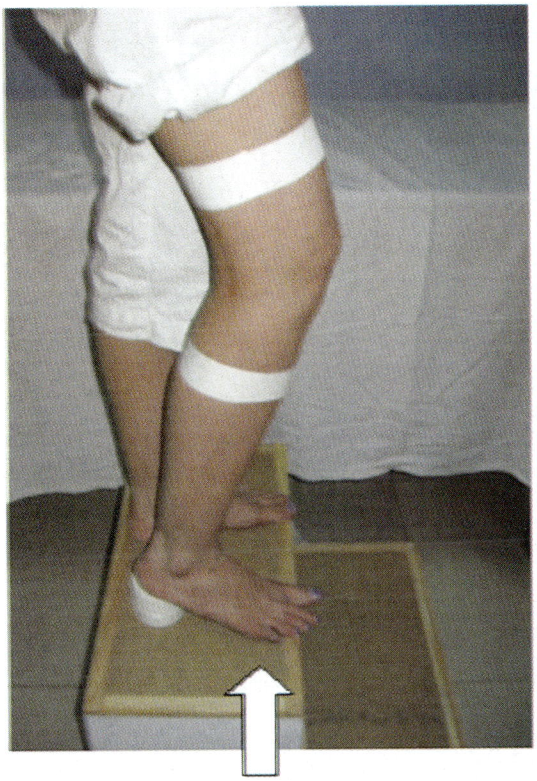

Fig. 8.4(b)

3. Begin the lateral (3 inch) elastic adhesive tape X with a strip starting anteriorly on the distal anchor, pulling up strongly around the tibia, and lateral to the patella finishing on the proximal anchor posteriorly.

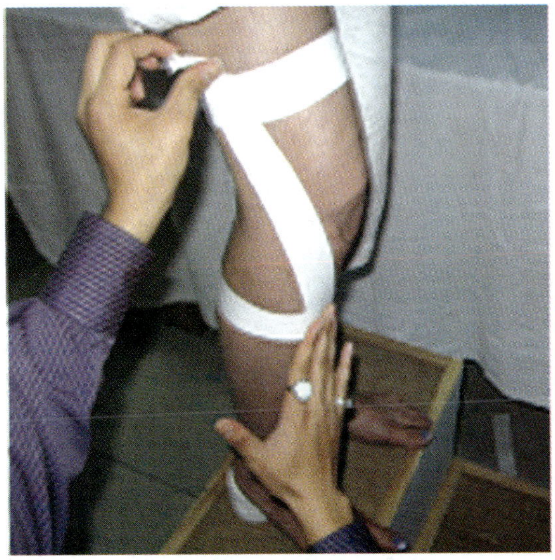

Fig. 8.4(c)

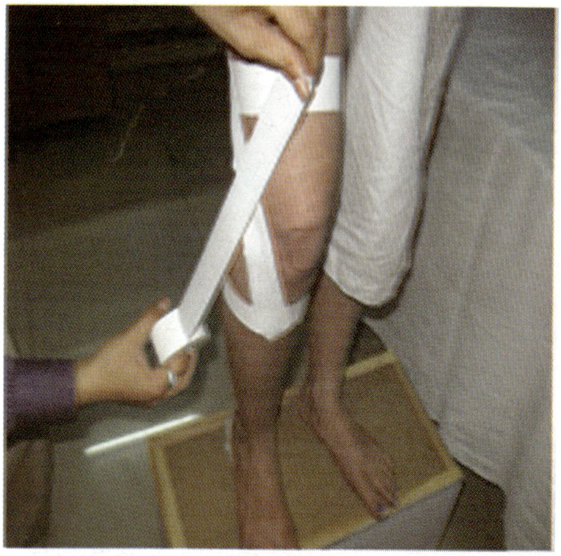

Fig. 8.4(d)

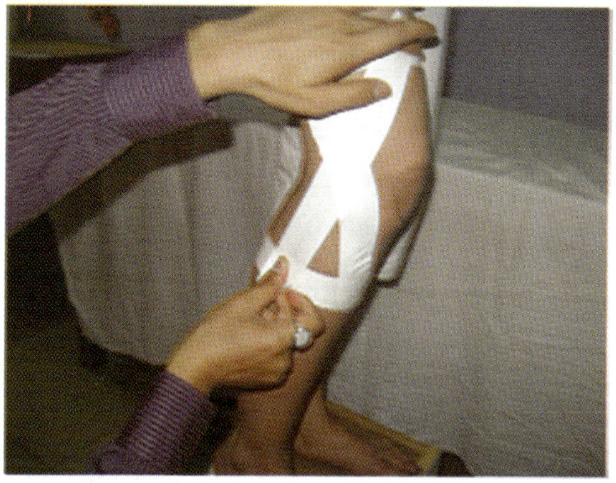

Fig. 8.4(e)

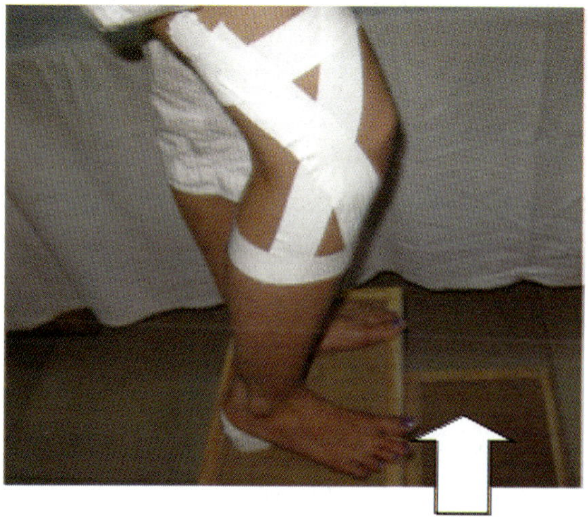

Fig. 8.4(f)

4. Complete the lateral X with a strip from the posteriolateral distal anchor, pulling up strongly to the anterio lateral proximal anchor, with the X over the lateral joint line.

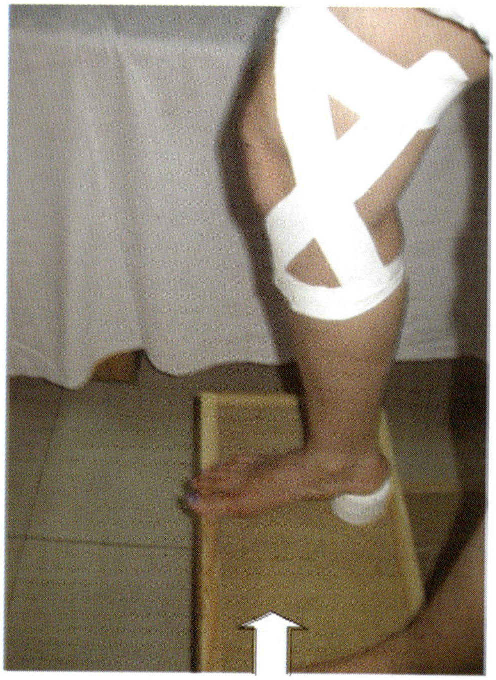

Fig. 8.4(g)

4. Repeat anchor X on the medial aspect without causing internal rotation of tibia or varus stress on the knee.

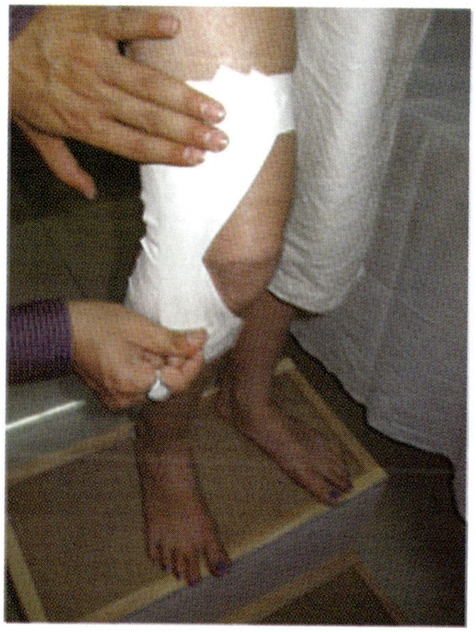

Fig. 8.4(h)

5. Use a vertical strip of white (2 inch) tape with the edges folded in for extra strength, to reinforce the lateral ligament. Start anteriorly on the inferior anchor, and pull up strongly on the lateral side, keeping the knee in maximum varus and adhere the tape securely to the proximal anchor posteriorly.

6. Complete this laterally reinforcing X with a second vertical strip starting posteriorly on the distal anchor, and crossing the previous strip at the joint line. Maintain maximal varus while adhering the end to proximal anchor anteriorly.

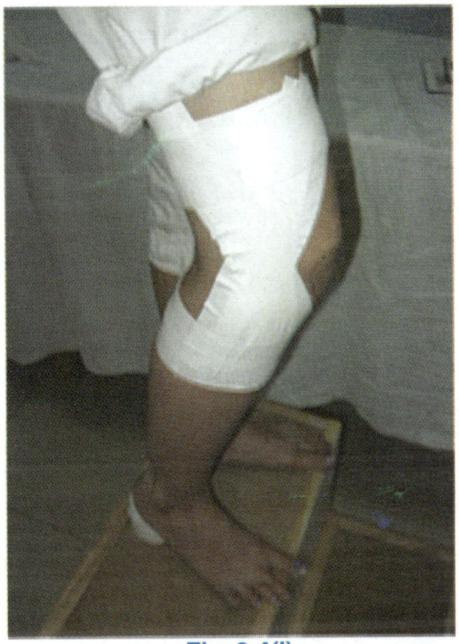

Fig. 8.4(i)

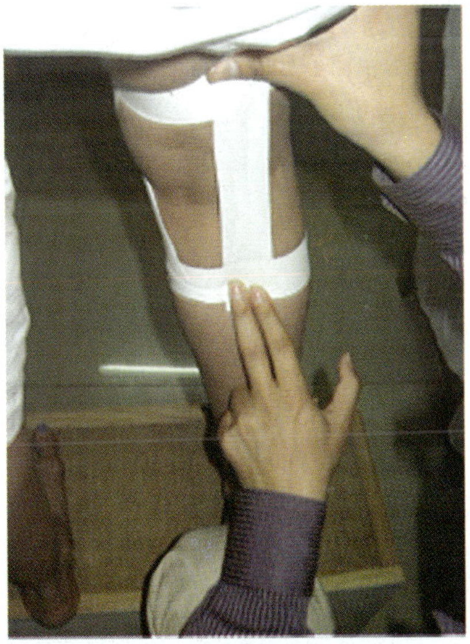

Fig. 8.4(j)

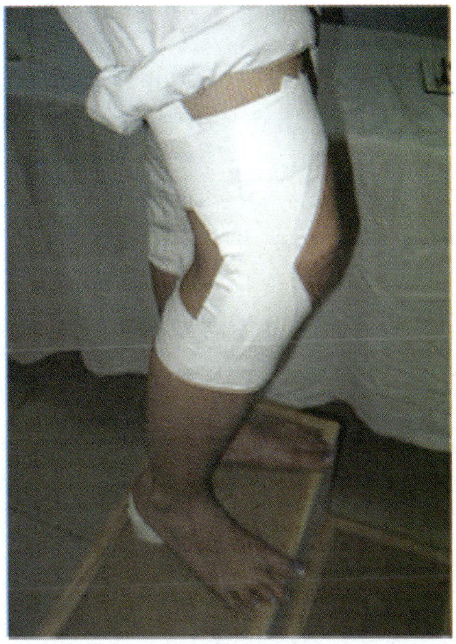

Fig. 8.4(k)

7. Apply a vertical strip posterior for more stability and reanchor at the proximal and distal aspect.

8. Before applying elastic wrap, test for degree of restriction:

   a. Extension must be restricted by 10 degree.

   b. There must be no lateral laxity, and

   c. There must be no pain on lateral stress testing (bending outwards) or extension.

NOTES:

- For acute sprains leave elastic wrap on for at least the first 48 hours.
- For back to sport taping, leave elastic wrap on for at least 15 minutes and remove for full activity.

TAPING FOR ANTERIOR CRUCIATE LIGAMENT (ACL) SPRAINS OF THE KNEE

Purpose

- Reinforces knee instability bilaterally and posteriorly.
- Prevents the last 20 degree of extension.
- Reduces anterior translation of tibia under femur.
- Allows almost full flexion and functional extension.

Indication for uses

- Anterior cruciate ligament sprains (acute, sub acute and chronic).
- Posterior capsular trauma.
- Hamstring strains.

NOTE:
- If an acute ACL injury is suspected the athlete must not return to field even if disability seems mild (in 3rd degree rupture, a "pop" is often felt).
- Be certain that the athlete is examined by a competent sport physiotherapist to confirm the diagnosis based on :
  a. A positive anterior drawer sign (forward sliding of the tibia under femur at 90 degree of knee flexion).
  b. A positive Lachman's test (forward gliding of the tibia at 20 degree of knee flexion).
  c. A positive pivot shift (sublaxations then sudden reduction of the lateral tibial plateau when flexing the knee from full extension with internal rotation of the tibia and a valgus stress at the knee).

MATERIALS

- Skin toughener spray.
- Razor.
- Pro wrap.
- Lubricant.
- Padding for hamstring tendons.
- (3 inch) elastic adhesive tape.
- (4 inch) elastic adhesive tape.
- (2 inch) Or (1.5 inch) non-elastic white tape.
- (6 inch) elastic wrap.

TERMINOLOGY

- Anterior cruciate ligament sprain: Severity of 1st to 3rd degree.
- Hyperextension injury.
- Torsion injury.

ETIOLOGY

- Forced anterior glide of the tibia under femur.
- Forced hyperextension.
- Forward fall with foot fixed in position.
- Direct frontal blow.

SYMPTOMS

- Often history of a "pop" sensation.
- Swelling.
- Active movement testing:
  a. Decreased range of motion and pain on end range extension, varying with severity.
  b. Decreased range and pain on extreme flexion is indicative of marked intra-articular swelling.
- Passive movement testing:
  a. Pain on end range extension with1st and 2nd degree sprains.
  b. Isolated 3rd degree may be pain free.
- Resistance testing (neutral position): No pain on moderate resistance.
- Stress testing: Positive "Lachman's" and lateral pivot shift test.

TREATMENT

Early

- R.I.C.E.S.
- Taping for ACL sprain taping.
- Therapeutic modalities.

NOTE: Surgery often recommended for 3rd degree of severity.

Later

Continued physiotherapy including:

- Therapeutic modalities.
- Avoidance of terminal knee extension initially.
- Specific strengthening of hamstring muscles.
- Gradual pain free returns to sport activity with taped support.
- Total rehabilitation program for range of motion, flexibility, strength and proprioception.
- May require bracing.

SEQUELAE

- Chronic pain.
- Instability.
- "Giving way"; "trick" knee.
- Predisposition to meniscal injury.
- Weakness of quadriceps.
- Degenerative arthritic changes.

POSITIONING

Standing on a stool or chair with a roll of tape under the heel of the injured leg and the knee in 40 degree of flexion (weight is borne on both legs).

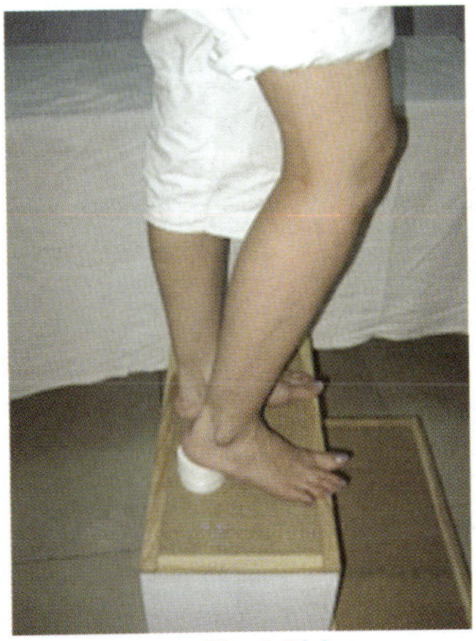

Fig. 8.5(a)

PROCEDURE (Figs. 8.5(a) to (m))

1. Clean, shave and dry the skin to be taped, checking for cuts, abrasions and sensitive areas.
2. Apply padding and lubricant to the popliteal fossa and hamstring tendons.
3. Apply skin toughener.
4. Apply prowrap and cover the area to be taped.

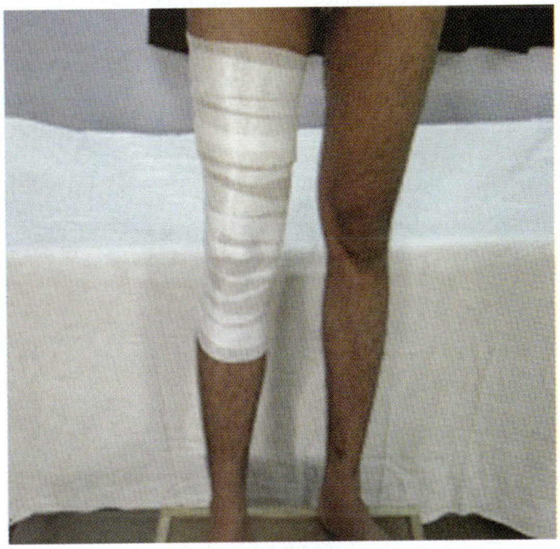

Fig. 8.5(b)

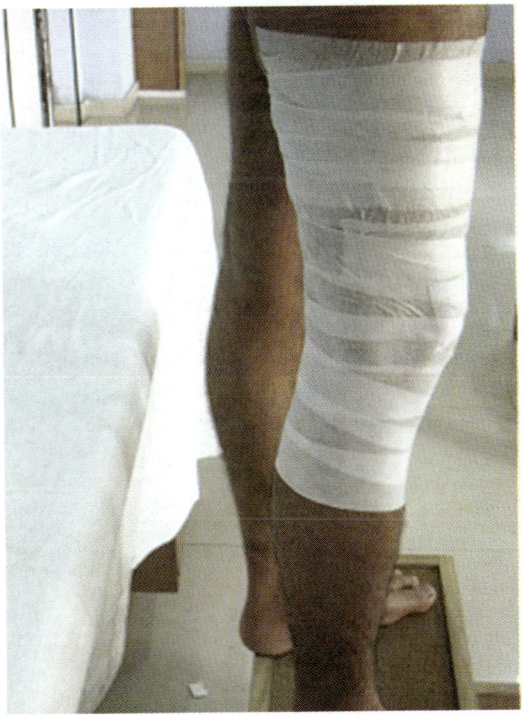

Fig. 8.5(c)

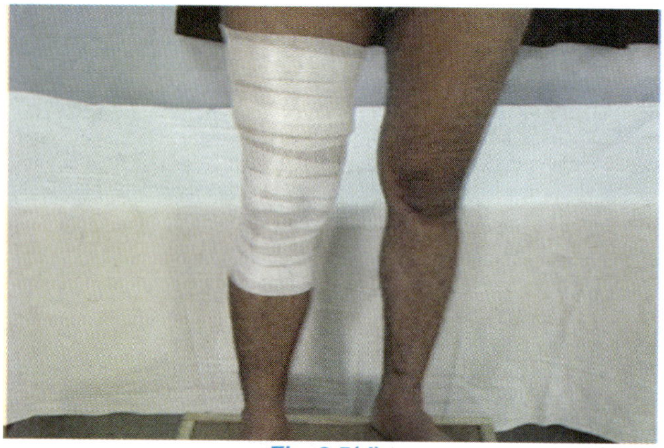

Fig. 8.5(d)

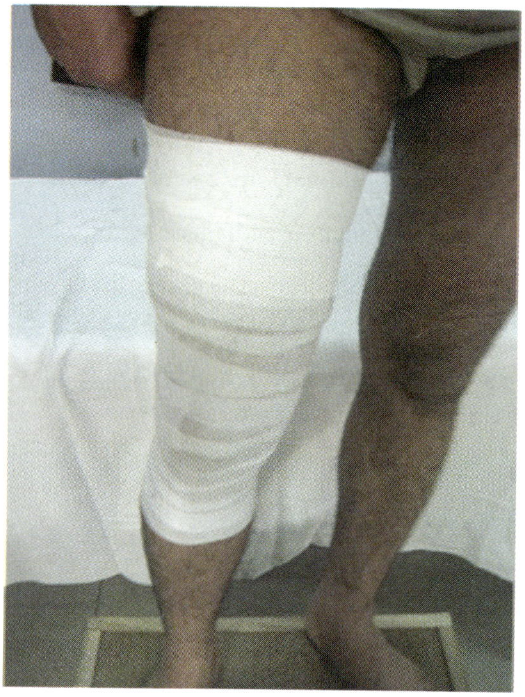

Fig. 8.5(f)

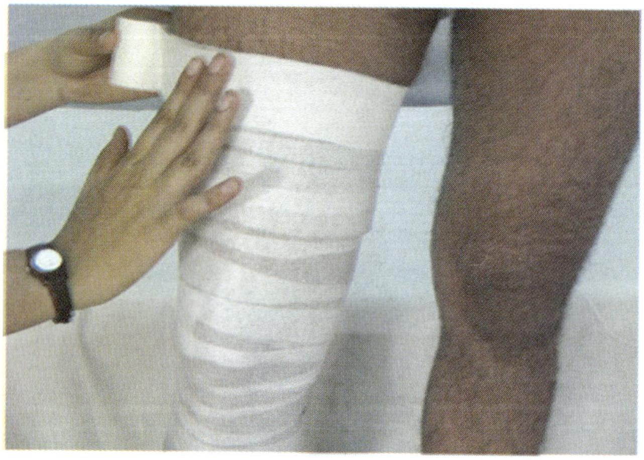

Fig. 8.5(e)

5. Apply proximal and distal anchors.

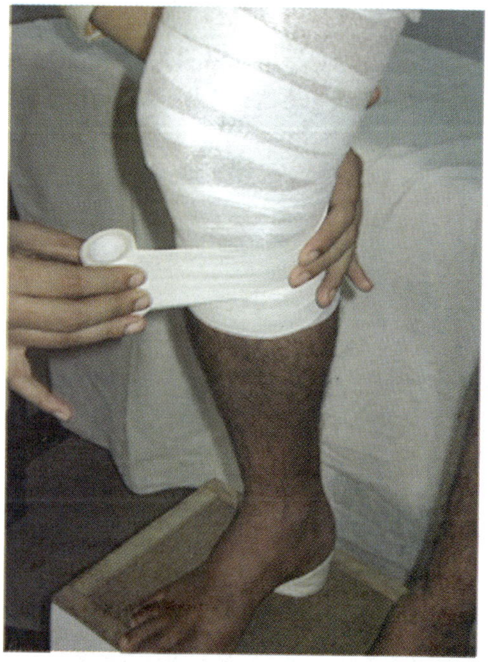

Fig. 8.5(g)

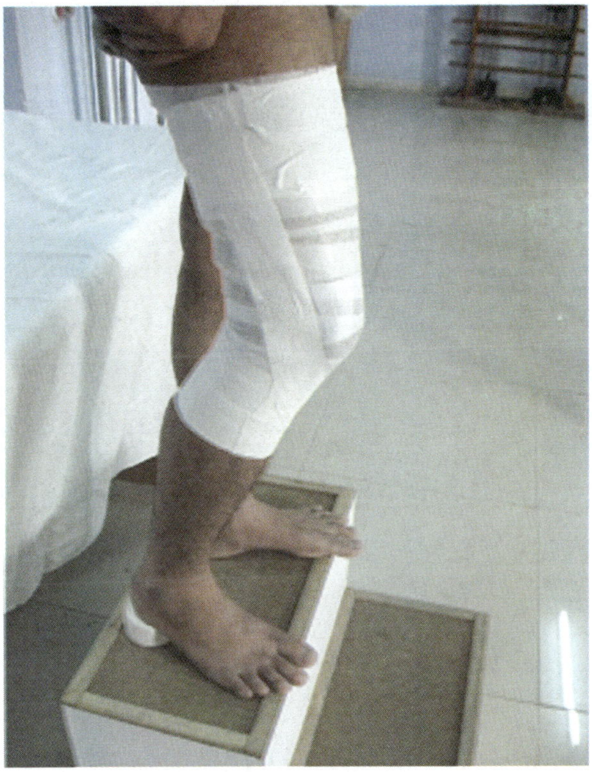

Fig. 8.5(h)

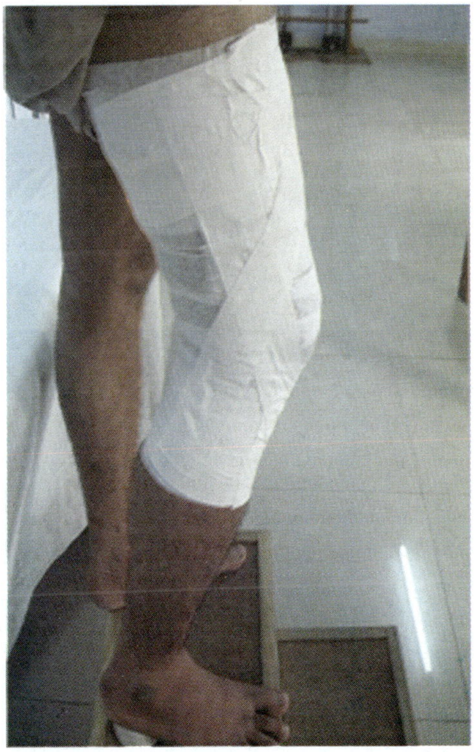

Fig. 8.5(i)

6. Apply (3 inch) elastic adhesive X over the medial joint line using moderate tension.

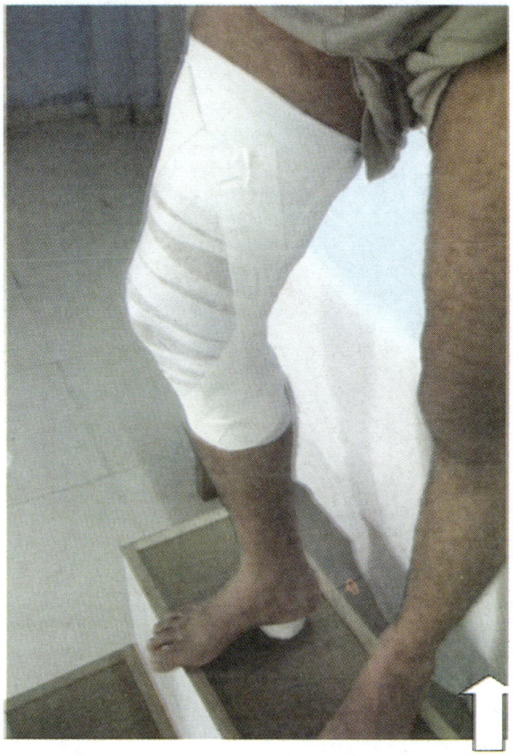

Fig. 8.5(j)

7. Repeat an X on lateral side.

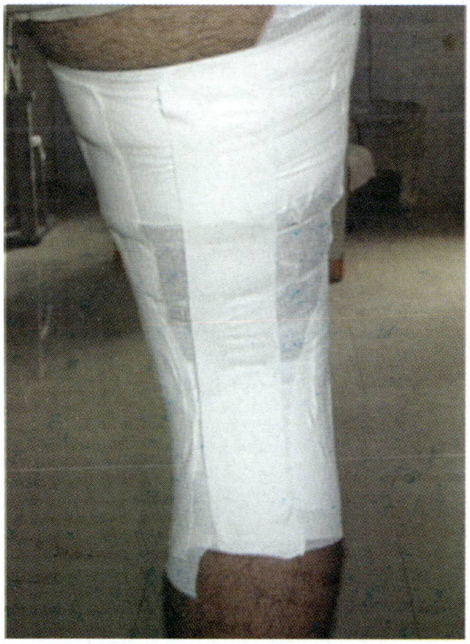

Fig. 8.5(k)

8. A vertical strip at posterior aspect for extra stability.

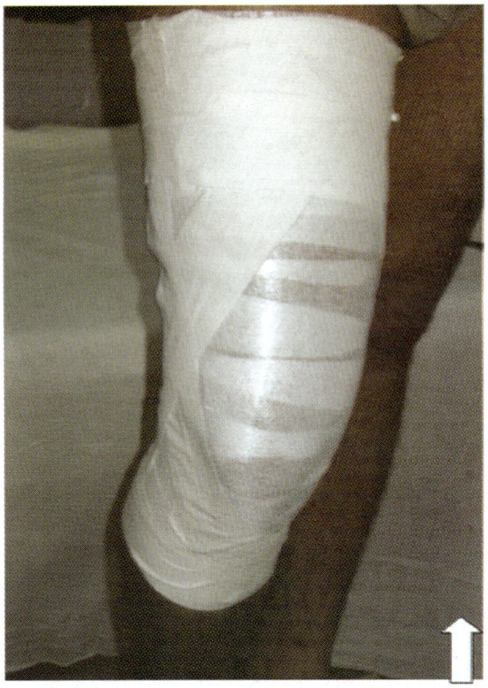

Fig. 8.5(l)

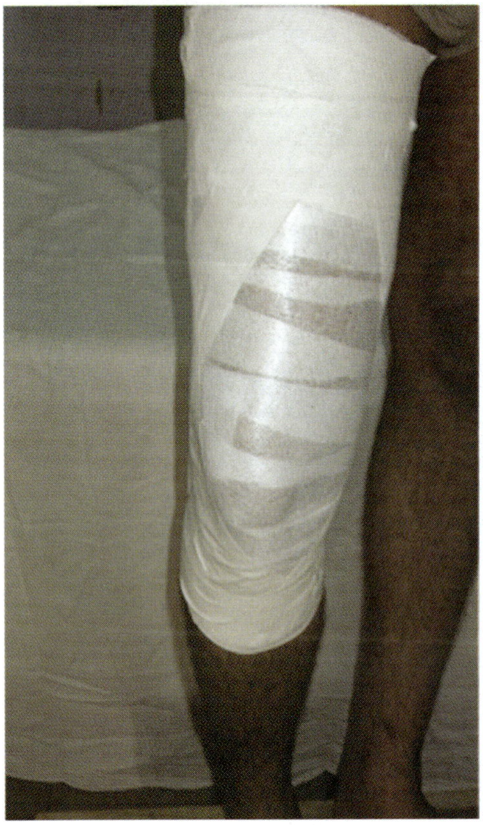

Fig. 8.5(m)

9. Reanchor these with (4 inch) elastoplasts from mid-thigh to mid-calf.

NOTE: Enough tension must be used so that the completed block at last.

10. Test the degree of restriction:
    a. Extension must be limited by at least 20 degree.
    b. There must a no pain on passive extension.

NOTE: Enough tension must be used so that the completed taping will completely block at least the 20 degree of knee extension when maximally stressed.

TAPING FOR PATELLO-FEMORAL PAIN

Purpose

- Compresses the patella tendon thereby changing lines of stress and thus altering the biomechanics of the patella-femoral joint.
- Reduces upward mobility of patella.
- Allow full movement at the knee joint.

Indication for use

- Patellar tendinitis.
- Patella-femoral pain syndrome.
- Osgood-Schlatter's disease.
- Medial knee pain associated with flat feet.
- "Jumpers knee".

NOTE:
- Evaluate pain on a scale of 0 to 10 with 0 being nil and 10 being the worst pain, prior to taping by having the athlete perform a half squat. Re-evaluate this movement throughout the taping procedure, monitoring any change in pain.
- Avoid compressing the patella against the femur, as this may aggravate pain.
- There should be no during activity, should the athlete not be function pain-free, McConnell techniques may be indicated.
- The semi-elastic adhesive tape used in this procedure is minimally adherent.

MATERIALS

- Razor.
- Quick drying adhesive spray.
- (1 inch.) semi-elastic tape (preferable) or non-elastic white tape.

(Semi-elastic tape: Has a minimal amount of elasticity and is not a conventional elastic adhesive tape).

TERMINOLOGY

- Patellar alignment syndrome.
- Retro-patellar inflammation.
- Pre-chondromalacia.

ETIOLOGY

- Quadriceps weakness.
- Poor tracking of patella.
- Subluxing or dislocating patella.
- Poor biomechanics of adjacent joint.
- Post traumatic blow to knee.
- Secondary to patellar tendinitis.
- Jumping as in plyometric training.
- Common in basketball and volleyball.

SYMPTOMS

- Peripatellar pain may be experienced in various locations:
  a. Diffuse around the patella (knee cap).
  b. At the inferior tip of patella.
  c. Anterior posterior to the patellar tendon.
  d. At the tibial tubercle (insertion of the tendon).
- Pain is often felt following sitting or resting.
- Active movement testing: May have pain on extension. pain when climbing or particularly when descending stairs.
- Passive movement testing: Muscle tightness or imbalance involving quadriceps, hamstring and tensor fascia lata (TFL).
- Resistance testing (neutral position): Weakness of quadriceps (specially vastus medialis oblique (VMO) with or without pain.
- Stress testing: Patella-femoral grinding test cause pain.

TREATMENT

Early

(If adequately inflamed)

- Ice.
- Therapeutic modalities.
- Lateral retinacular stretching.
- Taping: For patellar tendon taping.

Later

Continued physiotherapy including:

- Therapeutic modalities to control pain.
- Quadriceps re-education : Particularly vastus medialis obliqus [VMO].
- Utilizing muscle stimulation or biofeedback.
- Flexibility exercises, hamstring and tensor fascia lata (TFL).
- Gradually progressive negative weight training with corrected biomechanics (proper patellar tracking) and taping.
- Orthotics may help if faulty alignment is caused by poor foot biomechanics.

SEQUELAE

- Chronic pain of quadriceps.
- Weakness of quadriceps and later tensor fascia lata (TFL).
- Inflexibility.
- Inability to participate in sports.
- Chondromalacia.

POSITIONING

Relaxed, support long sitting position or supine, with the knee aligned in a neutral position and supported on a roll or cushion.

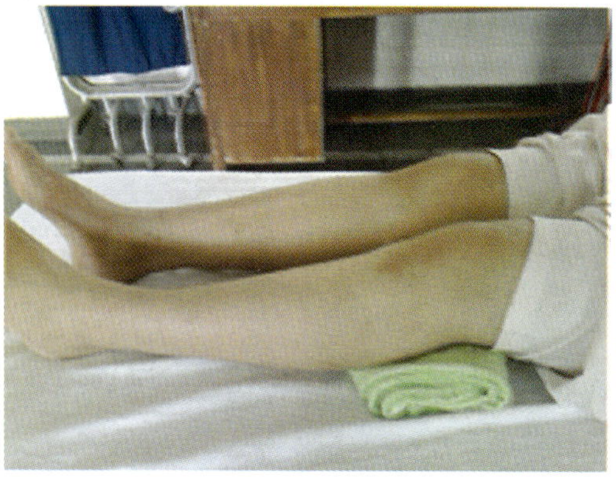

Fig. 8.6(a)

PROCEDURE (Figs. 8.6(a) to (h))

1. Clean, shave and dry the area to be taped, checking for cuts, abrasions and sensitive areas.
2. Spray liberally with quick adhesive spray and let dry completely.

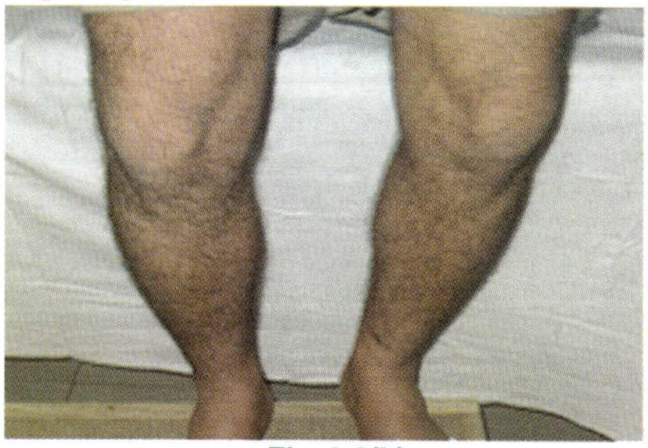

Fig. 8.6(b)

3. Perform the test position: A half-squat with weight more on the painful leg.

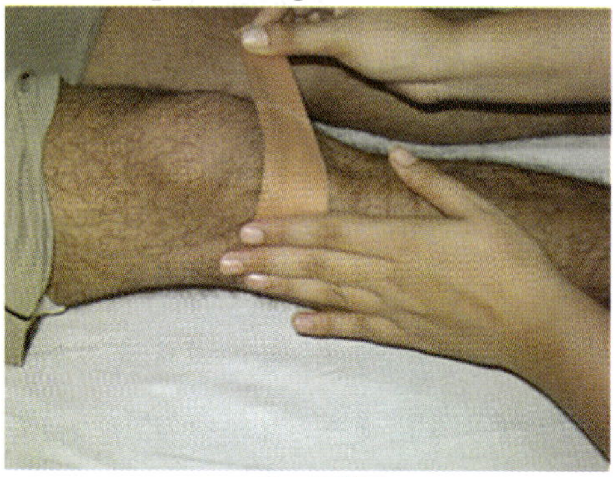

Fig. 8.6(c)

4. Starting posteriorly on the lateral side, apply a horizontal strip of (1 inch) semi-elastic adhesive tape. Using moderately firm pressure this strip should compress the patellar tendon just above the tibial tubercle.

NOTES:

- Do not encircle the leg completely.
- Make sure that the tape ends adhere well to the skin.

5. Re-evaluate the level of pain.

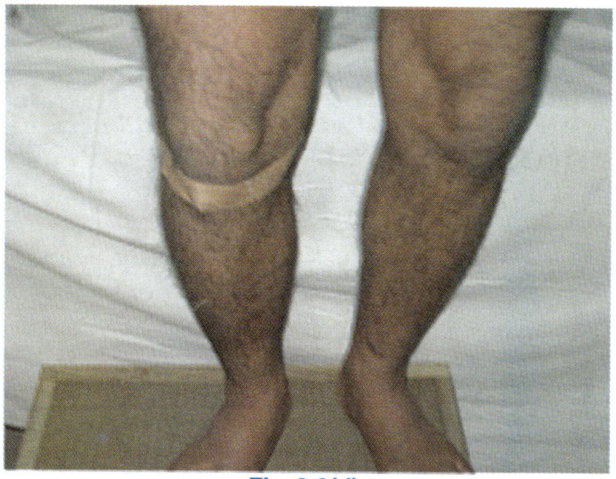

Fig. 8.6(d)

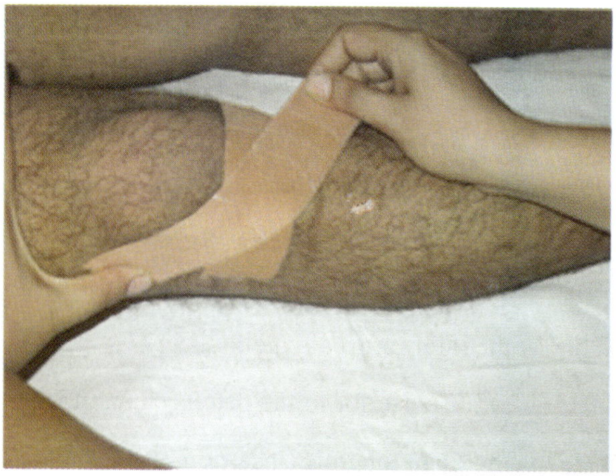

Fig. 8.6(e)

6. Apply a diagonal strip of tape from the upper lateral aspect of the knee beside the patella pulling distally across the patellar tendon ending medially.

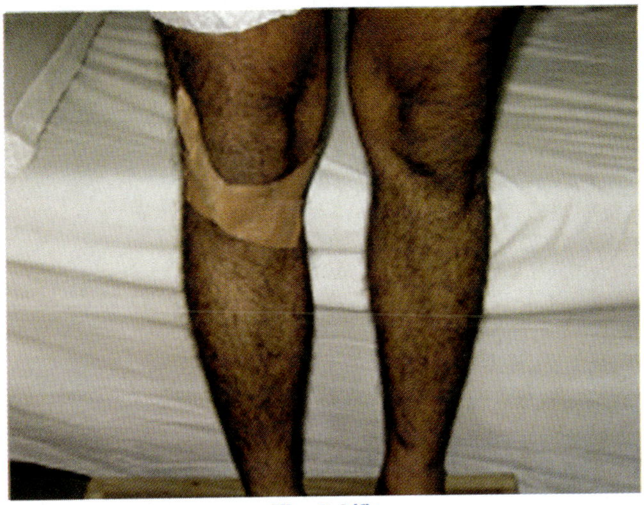

Fig. 8.6(f)

7. Re-evaluate the level of pain.

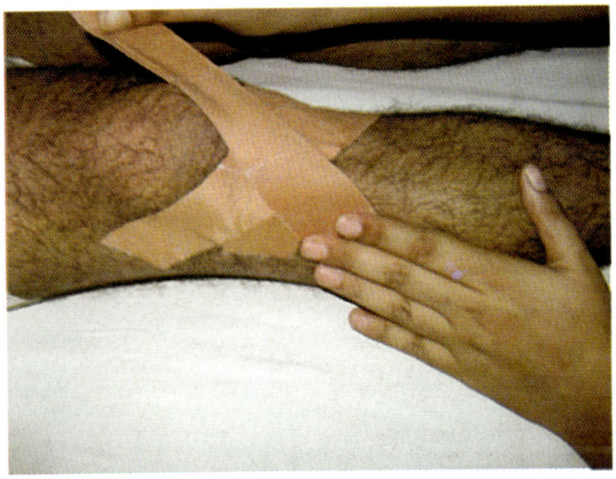

Fig. 8.6(g)

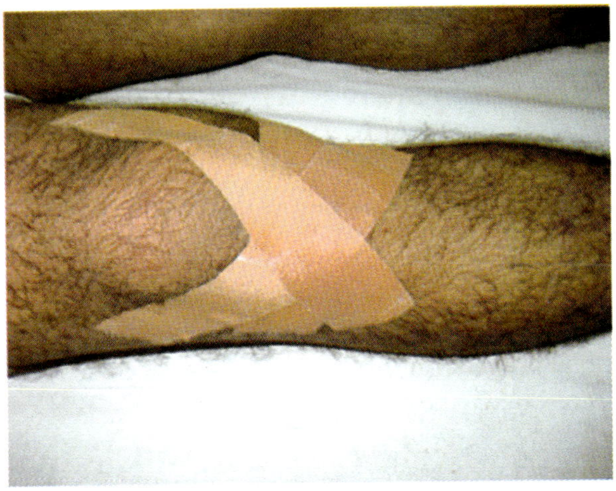

Fig. 8.6(h)

8. Apply a diagonal strip of tape from the lower lateral aspect of the knee beside the patella. Pulling proximally across the patellar tendon ending medially.

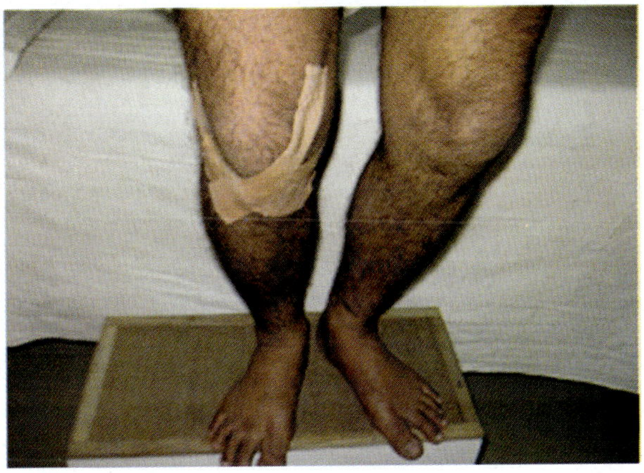

Fig. 8.6(i)

9. Re-evaluate the level of pain.
   a. 40 degree of full weight bearing flexion should be possible.
   b. If pain is not eliminated with the taping, try McConnell taping combined with biomechanically corrective approach.

NOTE:

Active physiotherapy should precede returning activity.

TAPING FOR QUADRICEPS (THIGH) CONTUSION OR STRAIN

Purpose

- Applies localized specific compression to the bruised or torn tissue.
- Prevents subsequent swelling, bleeding or muscle fiber tearing in the area.
- Allows for full function and stability.

Indications for uses

- Quadriceps contusion ("charley-horse").
- Quadriceps strain.
- For hamstring strains tape is applied to posterior thigh

NOTES:
- The exact site of contusion or strain must be localized.
- Pro-wrap is not recommended, as it significantly lessens the effectiveness of the tape technique.
- The pressure of the tape strips must be localized to the injured area and not too tight circumferentially. If constricted, hamstring and calf muscles may cramp; the athlete may feel that the leg is weak, stiff or heavy.
- Icing and gentle stretching of the injured muscle should start immediately.
- Any massage is contraindicated in the early stage as it may cause further internal bleeding and potential development of myositis ossificans.

MATERIALS

- Razor.
- Skin toughener spray.
- (4 inch) Elastic adhesive tape.
- (3 inch) Elastic adhesive tape.
- (1.5 inch) Non-elastic white tape.
- (6 inch) Elastic wrap.

TERMINOLOGY

- Contusion of one of the quadriceps muscle 1st to 3rd degree of severity.
- "Charley-horse".

ETIOLOGY

- Direct blow on thigh (a puck forcefully hitting the thigh in ice hockey; or a direct hit to the thigh in rugby or football).

SYMPTOMS

- Pain, tenderness over site of injury.
- Swelling and hematoma if not treated immediately.
- Active movement testing: Pain on active contraction of quadriceps.
- Passive movement testing:

  a. Pain on knee flexion.

  b. Worse with hip extension.
- Resistance testing (neutral position): Pain and/or weakness of quadriceps.

TREATMENT

Early

- Ice.
- Taping for compression.
- Early flexibility exercises enhanced by active contraction of hamstrings.
- Only; no over-pressure.
- Therapeutic modalities.
- Gentle activity with taped compression.

Later

Continued physiotherapy including:

- Therapeutic modalities.
- Strengthing exercises: Pain-free.
- Flexibility exercises.
- Gradual return to full pain-free activity with taped support. For compression taping.

SEQUELAE

- Hematoma.
- Myositis ossificans if managed early.
- Complete rupture of muscle if used too early.
- Weakness.

POSITIONING

Sitting on bench with knee flexed over the edge, and the heel resting on the ground floor.

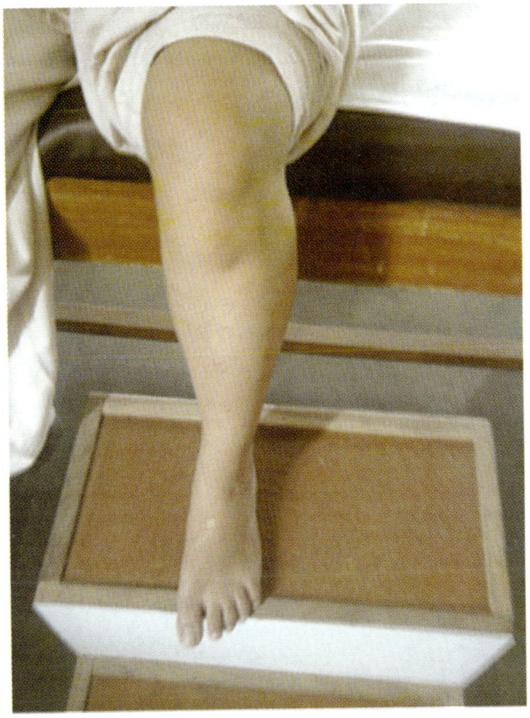

Fig. 8.7(a)

PROCEDURE (Figs. 8.7(a) to (e))

1. Clean, shave and dry the area to be taped, checking for cuts, abrasions and sensitive areas.
2. Localize and mark the exact site of the contusion or muscle strain.
3. Spray quick dry adhesive circumferentially to the thigh and let dry completely.

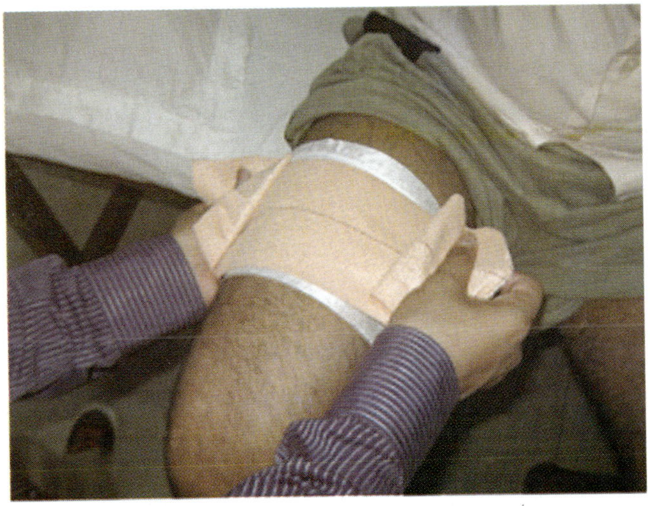

Fig. 8.7(b)

4. Begin (3 inch) below the lower aspect of the injury, wraps (4 inch) elastic adhesive tape around the limb using light tension.

NOTE: This layer of tape forms a foundation for the compression strips to avoid excessive tension on the skin.

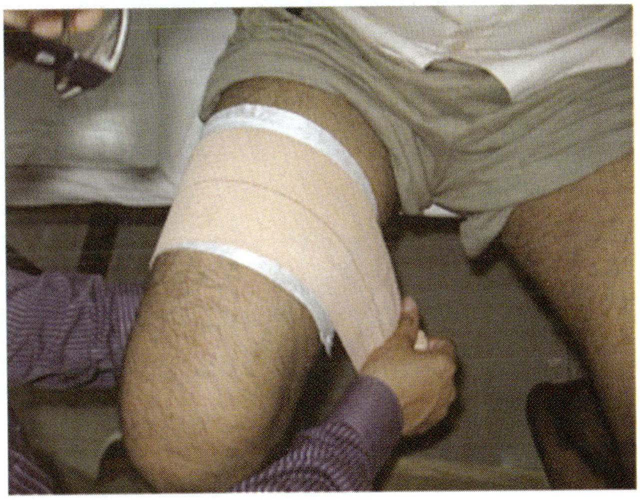

Fig. 8.7(c)

5. Apply strong pressure to the limb equally with both hands while maintaining lateral stretch until the tape reaches 3/4 of the way around the limb. Wrap the tape ends towards the back.

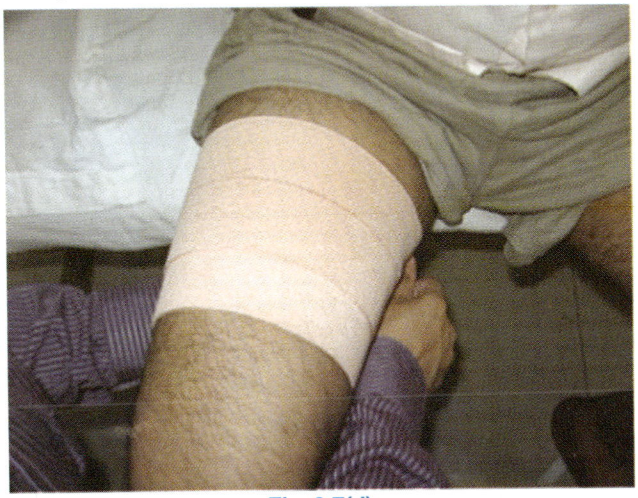

Fig. 8.7(d)

6. Complete encircling the limb by overlapping tape ends well at the back without tension.

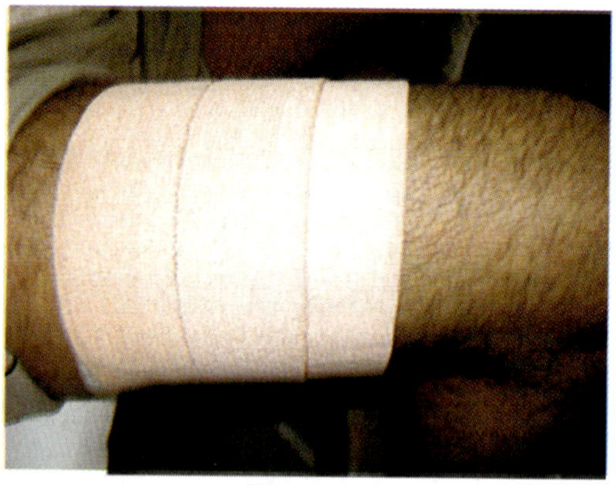

Fig. 8.7(e)

7. Wrap the entire tape job with an elastic wrap to activity, to give the adhesive in tape the time and heat necessary in order to set.
8. Affix the elastic wrap with white tape.
9. Reassess the degree of pain isometrically and dynamically.

9 Shoulder Taping

SHOULDER AND ELBOW

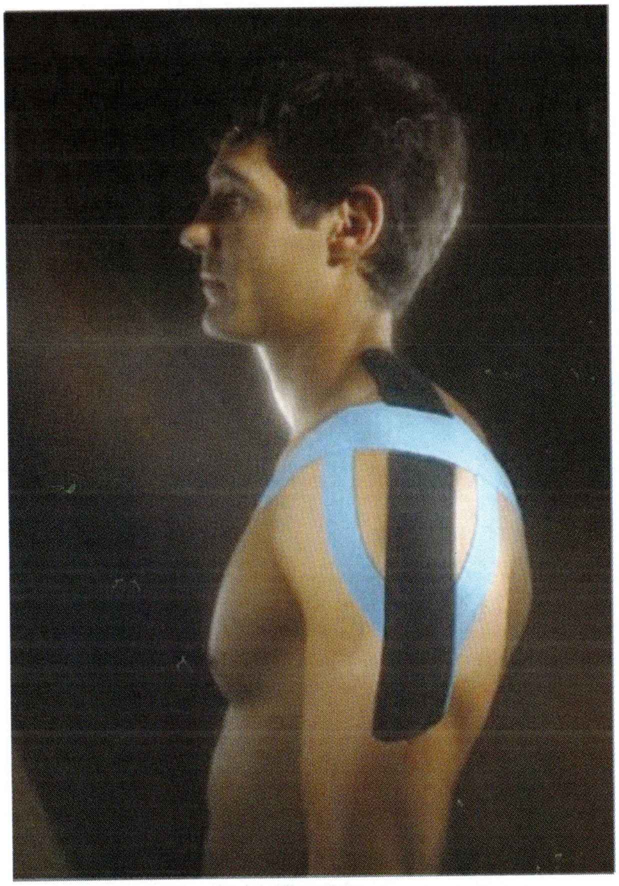

Fig. 9.1

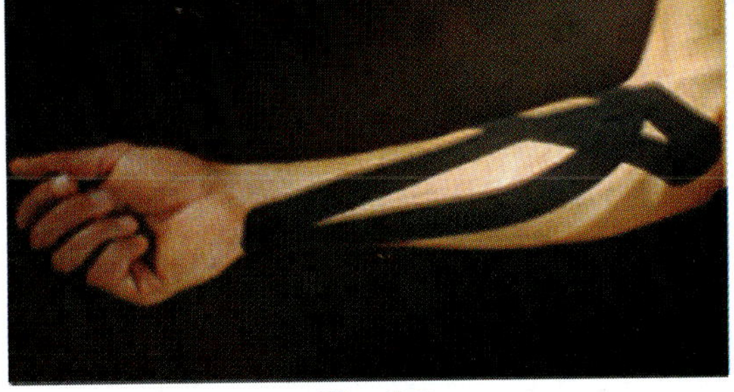

Fig. 9.2

The **gleno-humeral** (shoulder) joint is the most mobile of all the joints in the human body. It is this mobility that predisposes the shoulder to instability–both acute and chronic and heightens the joint's dependency on muscular and capsular support. By contrast the adjacent **acromio-clavicuar (A/C)** joint, is less mobile and depends solely on ligaments for support.

RIGHT SHOULDER FROM THE FRONT

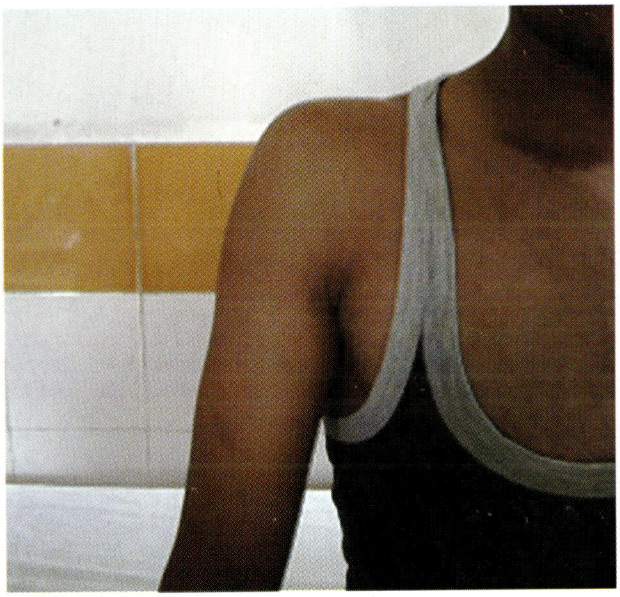

Fig. 9.3

The arm is slightly abducted:

- The nipple in the male normally lies at the level of 4th intercostals' space.
- The deltopectoral groove containing the cephalic vein is formed by adjacent borders of deltoid and pectoralis major.
- The lower border of pectoralis major forms the anterior fold.

MUSCLES PALPATION

1. Trapezius.
2. Deltoid.
3. Anterior process margin of deltoid.
4. Pectoralis major.
   - Upper margin of Pectoralis Major.
   - Lower margin of Pectoralis Major.
5. Biceps short head.
6. Coraco brachialis.
7. Teres major.
8. Serratus anterior.
9. Triceps.

TENDONS

10. Lattisimus dorsi.

BONES

11. Acromian of scapula.
12. Acromial end of clavicles.
13. Greater tuberosity of humerus.

JOINTS

14. Acromioclavicular.

HOLLOWS

15. Delto pectoral groove.
16. Supra clavicular fossa.
17. Infra clavicular fossa.

MISCELLANEOUS

18. Areola.
19. Nipple.

The right axilla or armpit is the hollow below the shoulder. Its anterior wall is made up mainly of fibers of pectoralis major with pectoralis major behind. The pectoralis wall consists of teres major with the tendon of lattisimus dorsi immediately in front. Close to pectoralis major a bundle of muscle made up of the short head of biceps and coracobrachialis runs down the arm with the cords of brachial plexus. Surrounding the axillary artery immediately behind. The axilla is also very important site for lymph glands draining lymphatic's from the arm and most importantly the breast.

MUSCLES

1. Trapezius upper fibres.
2. Trapezius middle fibres.
3. Trapezius lower fibres.
4. Deltoid.
5. Rhomboidus major.
6. Supra spinatus.
7. Infra spinatus.
8. Teres minor.
9. Teres major.
10. Lattisimus dorsi.
11. Triceps.

BONES

12. Spine of scapula.
13. Vertebral border of scapula.
14. Inferior angle of scapula.
15. Acromian process of scapula.
16. Acromial end of clavical.

NERVES

17. Axillary nerves posterior to humerus.

JOINTS

18. Acromioclavicular.

RIGHT SHOULDER FROM BEHIND

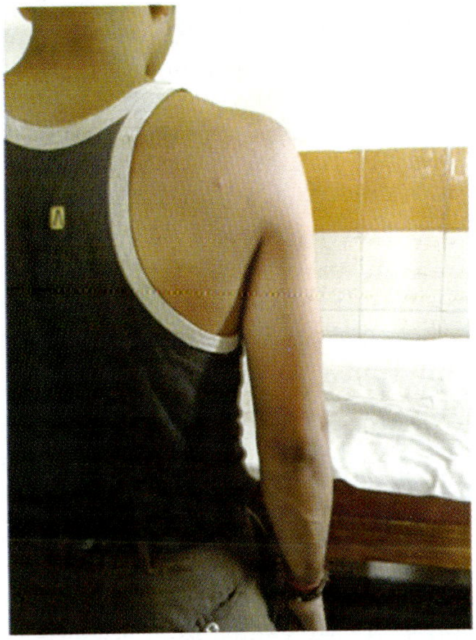

Fig. 9.4

The arm is slightly abducted and the inferior angle of scapula has been made to project backwards by attempting to flex the shoulder joint against resistance.

- The inferior angle of the scapula usually lies at the level of 7th intercoastal space. It is overlapped by the upper margin of lattisimus dorsi.
- The axillary nerve runs transversally under cover of deltoid behind the shaft of humerus at the level of 5 to 6 cm below the acromian.
- Lattisimus dorsi and teres major from the lower boundary of the posterior wall of axilla.

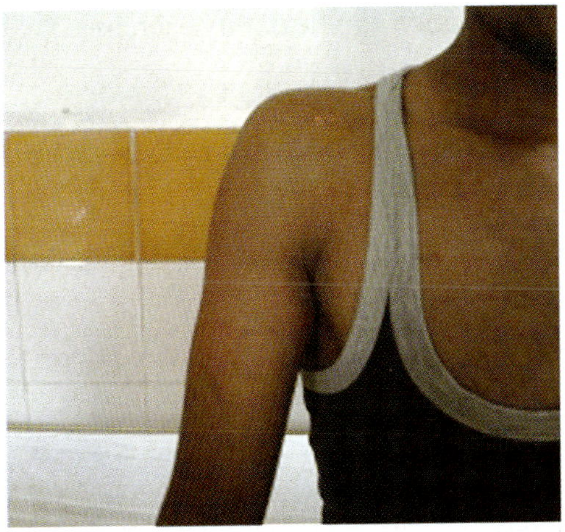

Fig. 9.5

RIGHT SHOULDER FROM FRONT

While maintaining good postural control of trunk the right arm has been abducted through some 180 degree. The left scapula remains in a normal resting position but with a firm muscle control, the glenoid pointing laterally. The right scapula has been rotated through some 70 to 75 degree under the activity of trapezius with the remaining arm movement occurring at the shoulder joint activity is obvious in deltoid the major abductor at shoulder joint, and no doubt in supraspinatus, through this muscle is marked by trapezius.

TAPING FOR ACROMIO-CLAVICULAR (A/C): SHOULDER SEPARATION

Purpose

- Compresses and stabilizes the acromio-clavicuar (A/C) joint.
- Keeps the distal end of the clavicle down while allowing almost full gleno-humeral function.
- Elastic support assist abduction.

Indications for use

- Acute A/C sprain.
- Sub-acute shoulder separation.
- Chronic shoulder separation.
- Chronic step deformity accompanied.

Tips: Ensure that step deformity is corrected/ reduced by proper positioning.

NOTES:

- Acutely injured athletes should not return to competition without proper investigation (high risk of advancing severity of the injury).
- Ensure correct diagnosis by following up with a sports-medicine specialist.
- Be certain that a radiological evaluation is done, particularly if any deformity is present.
- The taping can be used for a female athlete by applying the chest anchors below the breasts,

and the anterior end of the vertical anchor angled more toward midline.

- Monitor limb sensation, strength of pulse and various return prior to, during and after taping to ensure that there is no neuro vascular compromise.
- Tender skin at the axilla (armpit) need a special attention and protection.

MATERIALS

- Rectangular piece of felt or very dense foam.
- Approximately (2 × 1.4 inch) and 1 cm (0.4 inch) thick to cover A/C joint.
- Square of gauze, thin felt or folded prowrap.
- Approximately (2 inch, sq.) to cover nipple.
- Razor.
- Skin toughener spray.
- (1.5 inch) white tape.
- (3 inch) elastic adhesive tape.

INJURY: SHOULDER SPRAIN ACROMIO-CLAVICULAR (A/C) SEPARATION

TERMINOLOGY

- Sprains of acromio-clavicuar joint: 1st-3rd degree of severity.
- Shoulder separation.

ETIOLOGY

- Direct impact to the point of the shoulder.
- A fall; landing on the tip of the shoulder.
- A severe fall on the outstretched arm.
- Common in hockey, rugby, football, horseback riding and martial arts.

SYMPTOMS

- Pain and tenderness over the top of the acromio-clavicuar joint.
- Local swelling and bruising.
- Active movement testing, pain on all movements, particularly on flexion and horizontal adduction.
- Resistance testing: pain on all movements.
- Passive movements testing: Pain on horizontal adduction.
- Stress testing: varying degree of pain and step deformity between the clavicle and the acromian in 2nd and 3rd degrees of sprain severity.

TREATMENT

Early

- R.I.C.E.S.
- Taped support for A/C separation taping a sling can be offer additional support during first 48 hrs.
- Therapeutic modalities.
- 2nd and 3rd degree sprains should have at least three weeks of inactivity and support before dynamic treatment is started.

NOTE: Severe 3rd degree shoulder sprains may require surgery.

LATER

- Continued physiotherapy including.
- Therapeutic modalities.
- Range of motion and flexibility exercises.
- Strengthening: Isometric at first.
- Carefully guided progressive functional strengthening as tolerated.
- Gradual return to pain-free sports activity with taped sport.
- A felt donut over the joint can further protect it from impact in contact sports.

SEQUELAE

- Instability.

- Chronic pain.
- Associated strain of deltoid or trapezius muscles can cause residual weakness.
- Arthritic changes: Osteophyte formations.
- Clicking.

POSITIONING

Sitting comfortably with the elbow and forearm well supported across the lap with a solid cushion.

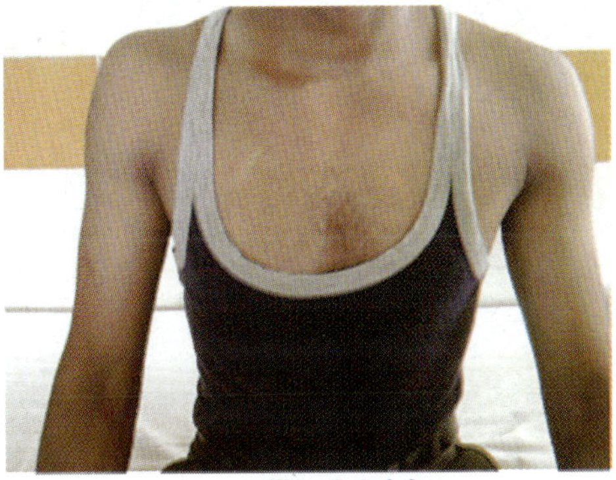

Fig. 9.6 (a)

PROCEDURE (Figs. 9.6(a) to (z))

1. Clean skin thoroughly and check for any abrasions, cuts, or sensitive areas.
2. Shave the upper arm and chest area in a (6 inch) strip.

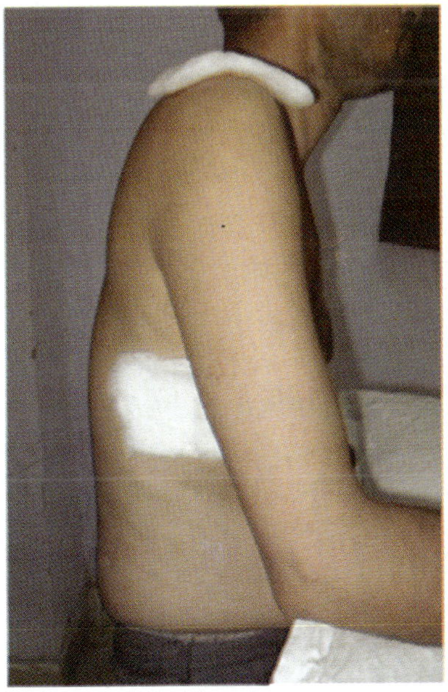

Fig. 9.6 (b)

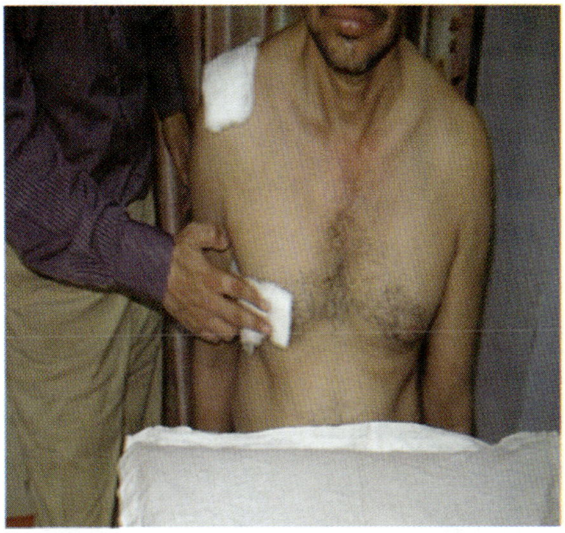

Fig. 9.6 (c)

NOTE: Sensation, pulse, temperature and colour must be checked before starting to tape.

3. Spray the area well with tape adherent to maximize adhesiveness thus stabilizing anchor.

Tips: Turn athletes face away and protect nipple when spraying.

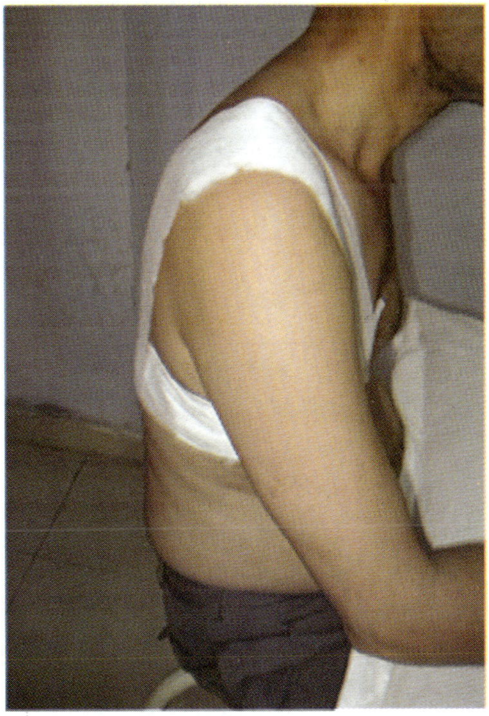

Fig. 9.6 (d)

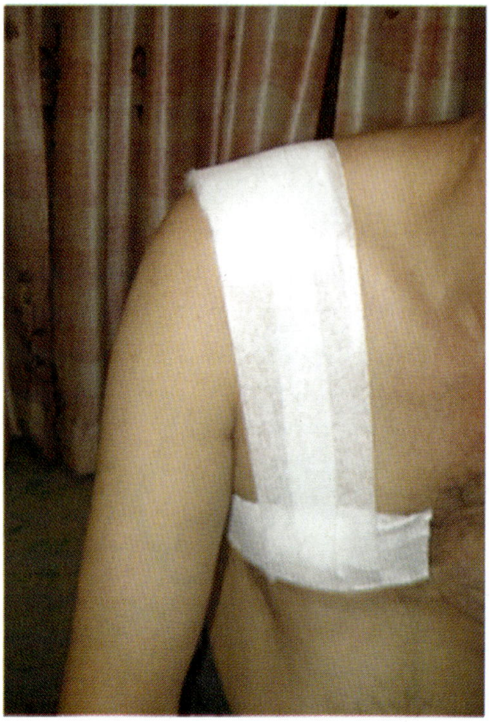

Fig. 9.6 (e)

4. Wrap an anchor with light tension around the mid humerus with (3 inch) elastic adhesive tape.
5. Apply two anchors of (3 inch) elastic adhesive tape horizontally to the chest with the light pressure from anterior to posterior at the level of fifth rib (covering the nipple with gauge, prowrap or felt).

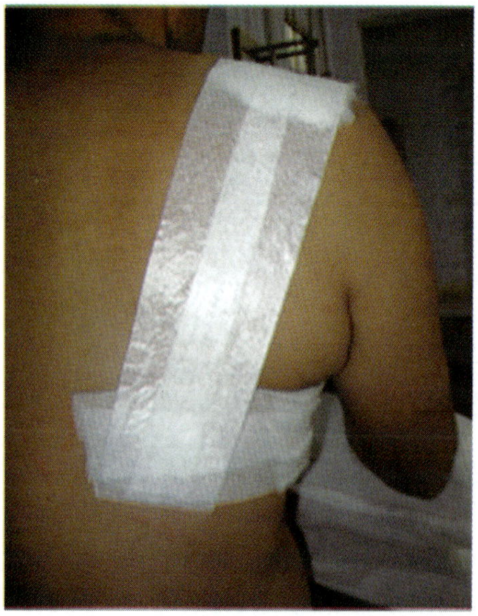

Fig. 9.6 (f)

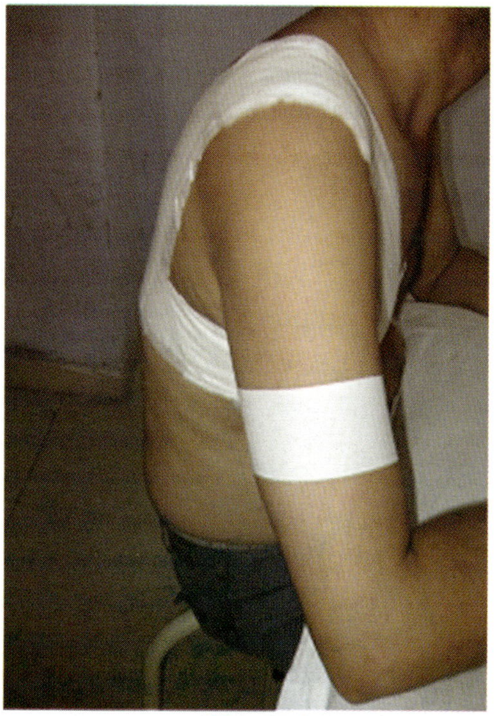

Fig. 9.6 (g)

Tips: Ensure that the last 7.5 cm (3 inch) the ends of the anchors are applied without tension and pressed firmly to avoid peeling back of the tape.

6. Cut the piece of felt or dense form padding large enough to cover the prominence of the A/c joint (approx.1.5 × 2 inch and at least 1 cm (0.4 inch thick).

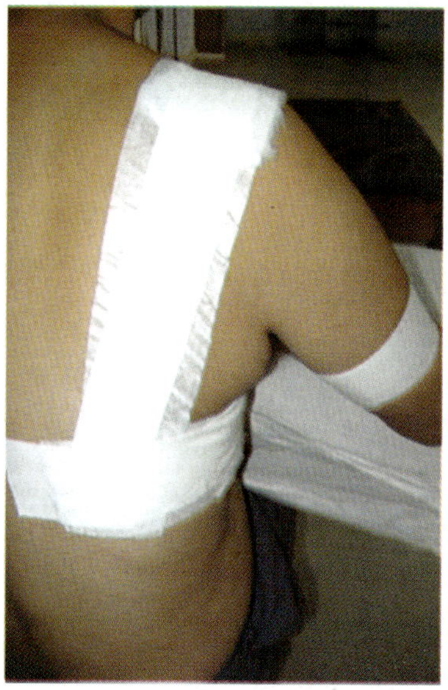

Fig. 9.6 (h)

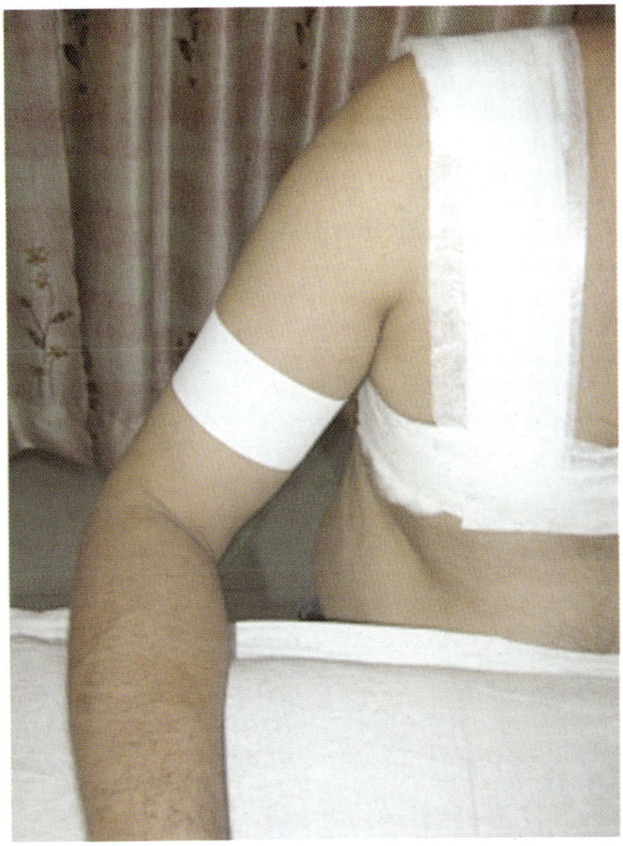

Fig. 9.6 (i)

7. Using (3 inch) elastic adhesive tape and moderate tension, apply rectangle directly on the upper end of the A/C joint (outer tip of the clavicle and adjacent acromian).

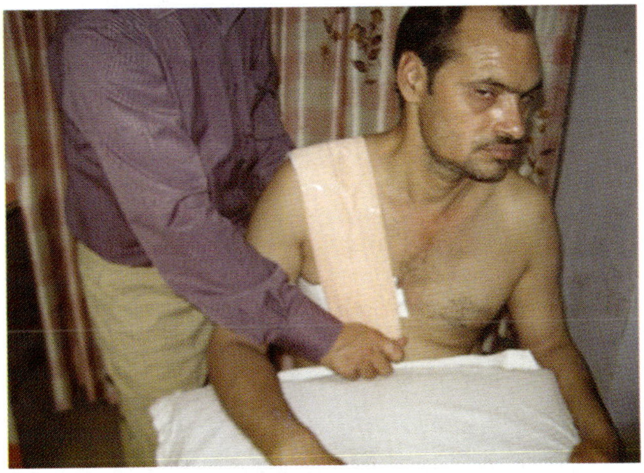

Fig. 9.6 (j)

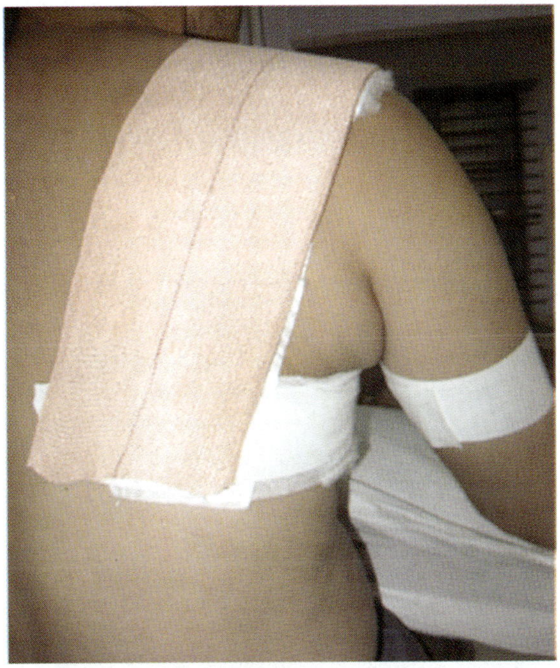

Fig. 9.6 (k)

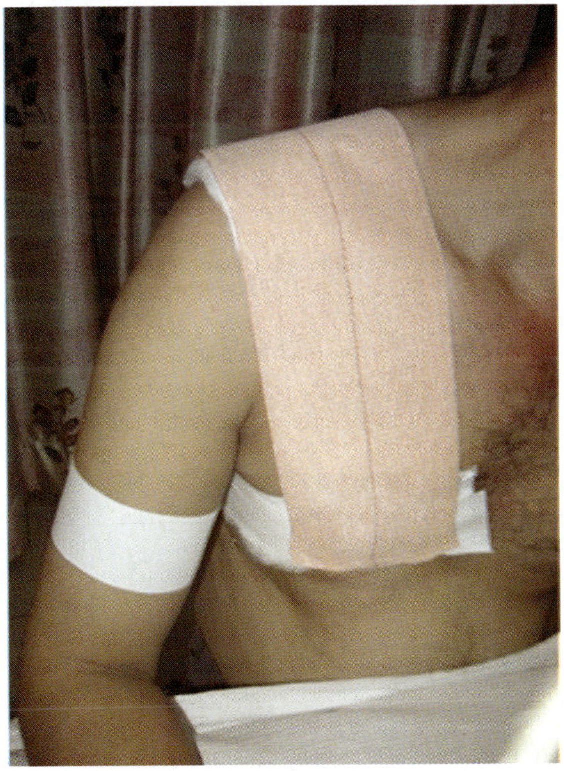

Fig. 9.6 (l)

8. Apply the compression strip of tape directly downward over the distal end of the clavicle. Extend the elastic tape horizontally as much as possible and

apply through the padding with strong pressure downwards while maintaining the horizontal tension. Release the tension when the end of the strip reach the chest anchors anteriorly and posteriorly (front and back).

9. Repeat this strip, moving laterally to cover one half of the first strip.

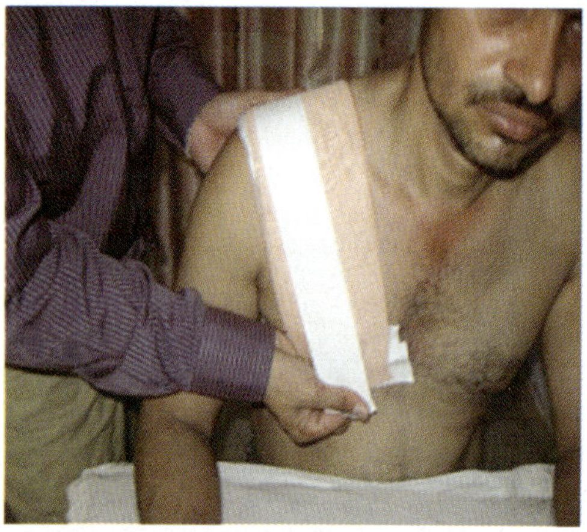

Fig. 9.6 (m)

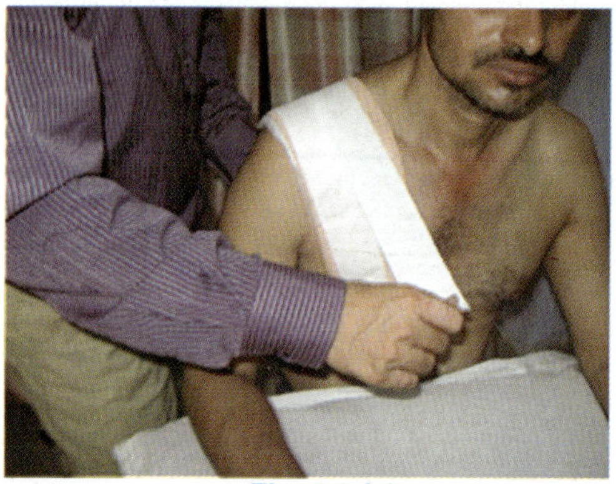

Fig. 9.6 (n)

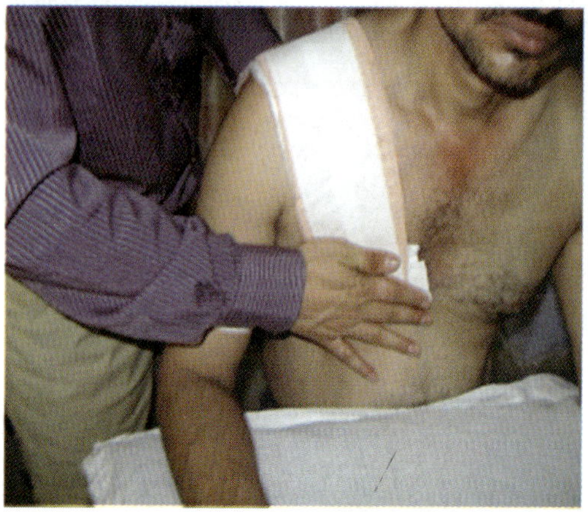

Fig. 9.6 (o)

10. Reinforce stability by applying a strip of (1.5 inch) white tape.
    (a) Maintain strong horizontal tension while applying strong pressure downward on the superior (upper) aspect of the A/C padding.
    (b) Ensure that these strip cross the anchors completely.

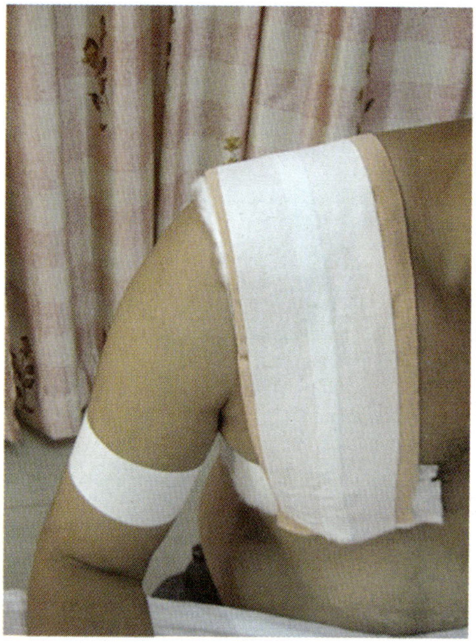

Fig. 9.6 (p)

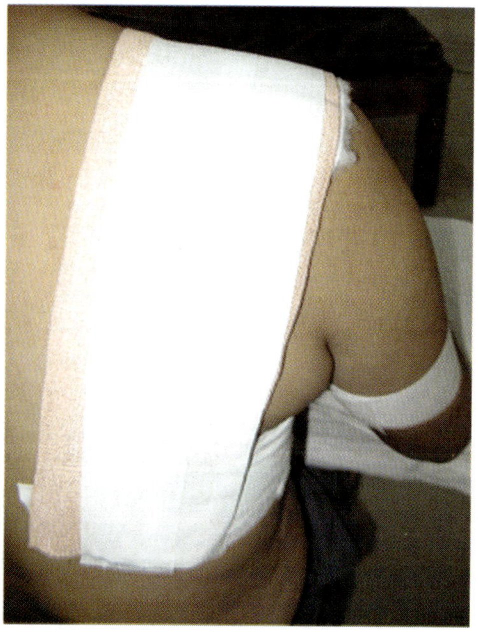

Fig. 9.6 (q)

11. Apply a second downward strip of white tape more laterally.

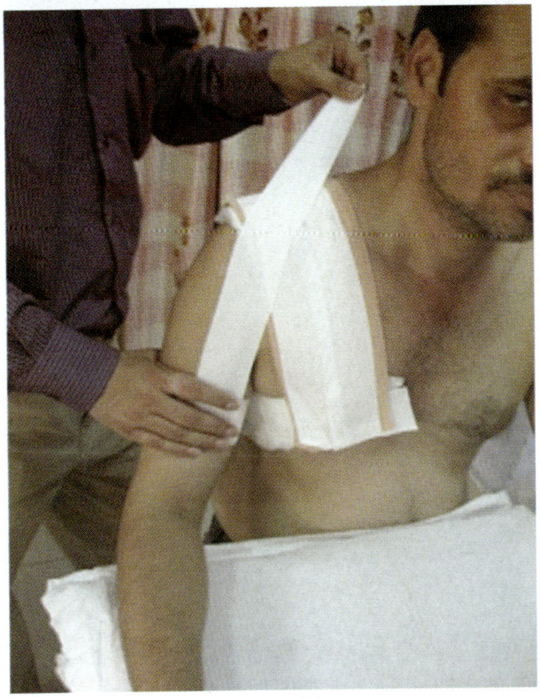

Fig. 9.6 (r)

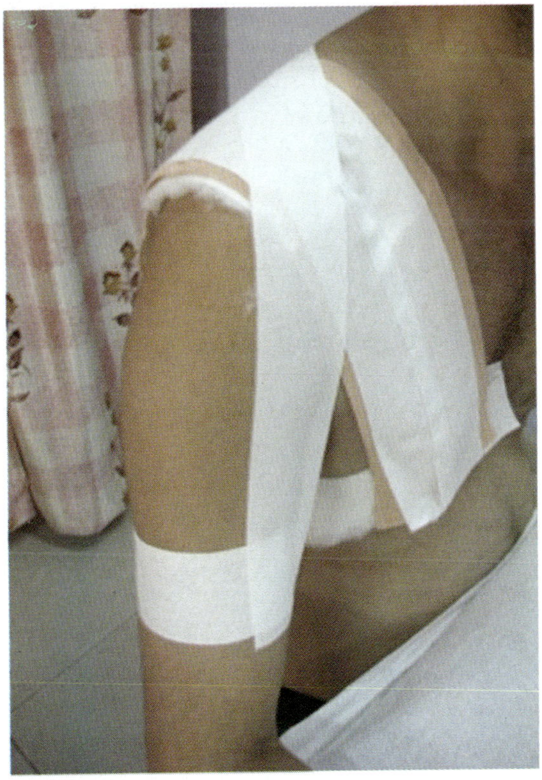

Fig. 9.6 (s)

12. With the arm in a 45 degree angle of abduction, place a strip of (3 inch) elastic adhesive tape starting laterally from the anchor going anteriorly across the top of the padding pulling up with firm tension to take the weight of the arm off the distal part of the joint.

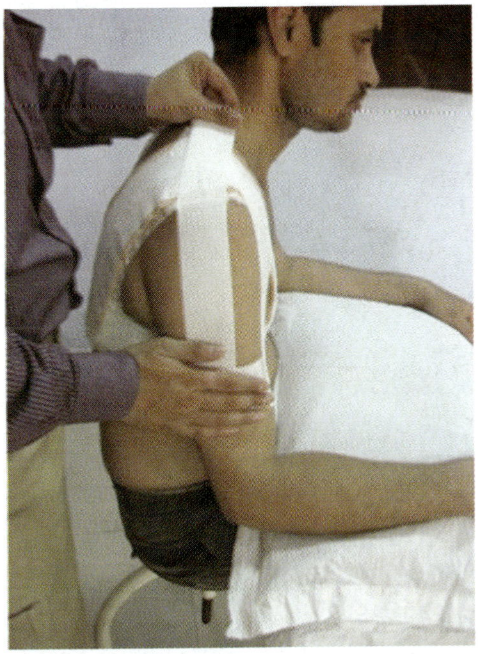

Fig. 9.6 (t)

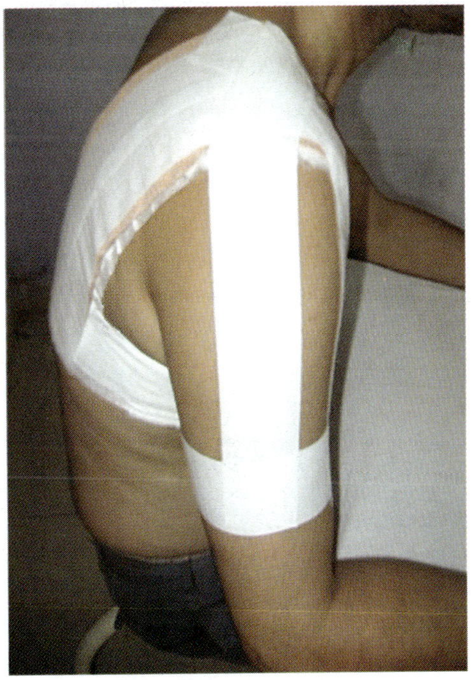

Fig. 9.6 (u)

13. Repeat this strip starting posterolaterally on the arm and pulling up on the posterior aspect of the deltoid muscle.

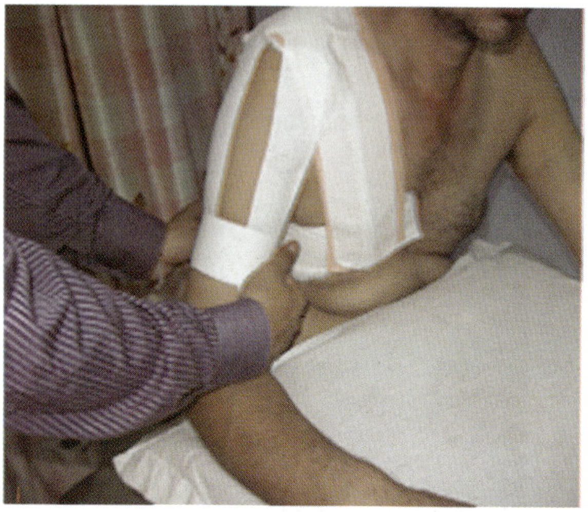

Fig. 9.6 (v)

14. Anchor the top of these last two strips with strip of elastic adhesive tape.

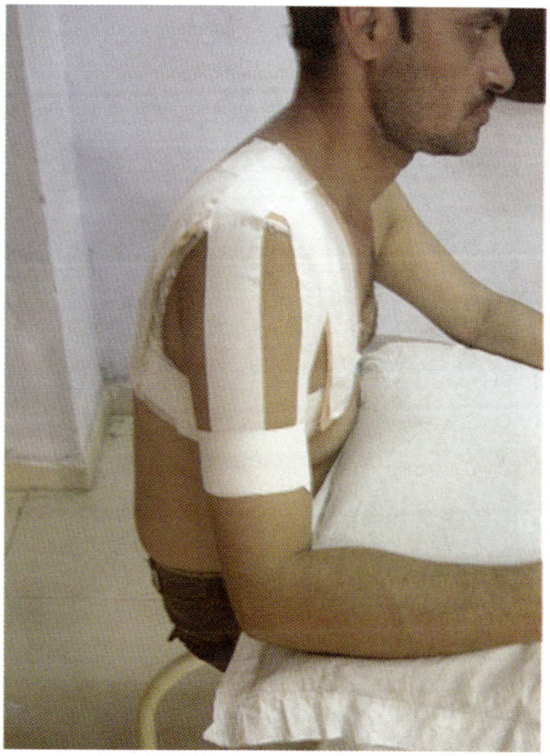

Fig. 9.6 (w)

15. Re-apply the humeral (arm) anchor strip.

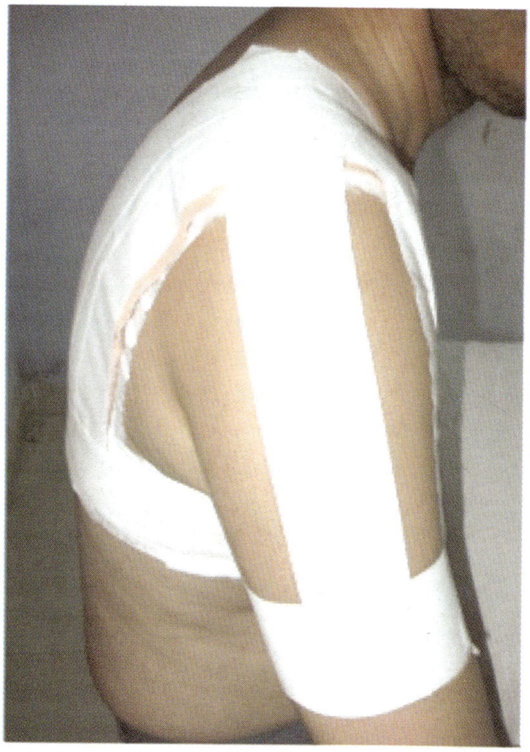

Fig. 9.6 (x)

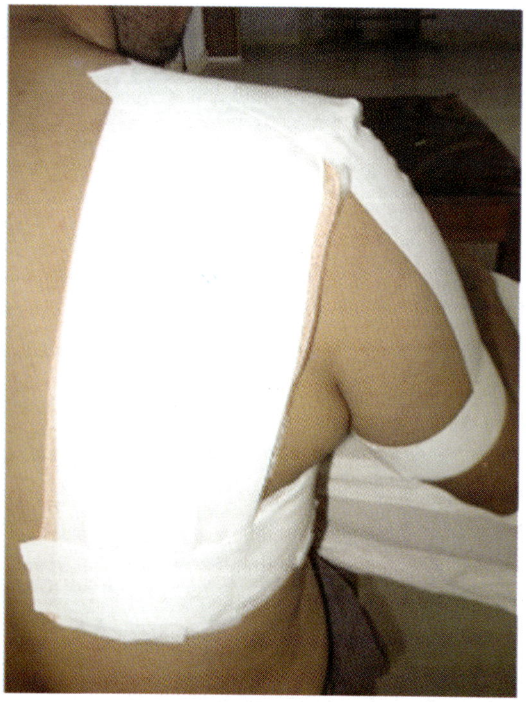

Fig. 9.6 (y)

16. Lateral and posterior view of finished taping.

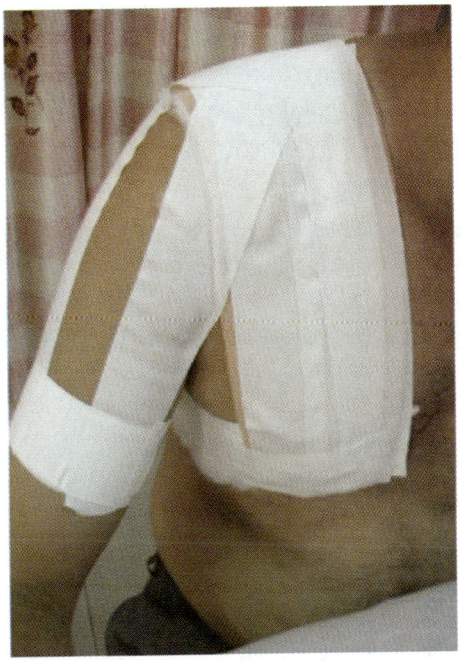

Fig. 9.6 (z)

17. Finish with a strip of elastic adhesive tape applies as the horizontal anchors to the chest to fix the lower end of the vertical strips of the tape.
18. Assess the degree of pain reduction post taping. Static and with unassisted arm flexion and abduction.

TAPING FOR GLENO-HUMERAL (SHOULDER) DISLOCATION/ SUBLUXATION

Purpose

- Prevents elevation.
- Severely limits possible abduction external rotation and flexion of the shoulder.
- Allows relatively functional range of motion below the plane of 90 degree.

Indications for uses

- Sub-acute shoulder subluxations.
- Chronic subluxations.
- Sub-acute shoulder dislocations.
- Apprehension in a previously or frequently injured athlete.

NOTE: This taping technique is not intended for acute dislocation of the shoulder.

Tips:

- Be certain that the correct diagnosis has been made in order to determine correct treatment.
- For repeat injuries check for possible axillary nerve damage: Deltoid weakness (abduction at 90 degree) and lateral shoulder numbness.
- Check that X-ray were taken after initial injury.
- Check stability tests for different types of chronic subluxations/dislocations:

1. ANTERIOR:

- Positive "apprehension test" (muscle guarding when shoulder is passively externally rotated at 90 degree of abduction).
- Anterior instability on the "load and shift test": Excessive anterior gliding of the humeral head when pressed forward while stabilizing the scapula (athlete sitting).

2. INFERIOR:

- Inferior instability: Longitudinal traction causes an inferior displacement and a palpable sulcus (hollow) as the tip of acromian (athlete sitting or lying).

3. POSTERIOR:

- Posterior instability or "clicking": When returning to a neutral position, after over-pressure is applied to a flexed and internally rotated shoulder (athlete sitting).
- Posterior instability on the "load and shift test": Excessive posterior gliding of the humeral head when pressed backwards while stabilizing the scapula (athlete sitting).

TERMINOLOGY

- 3rd degree sprain of gleno-humeral joint.
- Shoulder dislocation: Anterior or posterior.

ETIOLOGY

- Forced external rotation plus abduction of shoulder in varying degrees of elevation or a direct blow to the posterior aspect of the shoulder usually cause anterior dislocation.
- A fall on tip outstretched hand or a direct blow or fall on the anterior aspect of the shoulder can cause a posterior dislocation.
- Partial anterior dislocation (subluxations) is quite common contact and collision sports, when the athlete's arm is caught out from the side (abduction) with the hand upwards (external rotation).
- Chronic subluxations are common among athletes who perform repetitive movements at high speed at the outer reaches of their range of motion (such as baseball pitchers) or with great force (such as competitive swimmers).
- Common injury in the following sports: Hockey, football, baseball, basketball, wrestling, rugby, gymnastics.

SYMPTOMS

- Athlete feels shoulder has "popped out".
- A solid bulge either anteriorly or posteriorly.
- Hollow drop at tip of acromian.
- Active movement testing: Extreme pain and inhibition of all movements.
- Resistance testing (neutral position): Pain in all directions.
- Inability to actively contract biceps and deltoid muscles.
- Passive movement testing: Extreme pain on attempted passive internal or external rotation and abduction.

TREATMENT

Early

- R.I.C.E.S.
- Reduction by an experienced professional.

  Immobilization: Forearm should be strapped to chest wall for first three weeks before progressing to more dynamic treatment.
- Therapeutic modalities.

NOTE: Surgery is often indicated for extreme damage including avulsions, fractures, chip and nerve or vascular injury.

Later

- Continued physiotherapy including.
- Therapeutic modalities.
- Isometric strengthening.
- Progressive range of motion and flexibility exercise avoiding external rotation.
- Specific strengthening of internal rotators and adductors.
- Gradual return too activities with taped support.
- Full rehabilitation program to regain strength and coordination: Muscles stimulation or biofeedback are helpful.

SEQUELAE

- Recurrent dislocations.
- Permanently lax capsule.
- Weakness of shoulder rotators.
- Imbalance: Abnormal coordination of shoulder girdle musculature.
- Arthritic changes.

POSITIONING

Sitting with hand resting comfortably on the ipsilateral thigh, and the elbow positioning sideways. This position keeps the shoulder in internal rotation. Ensure that the elbow does not fall backwards.

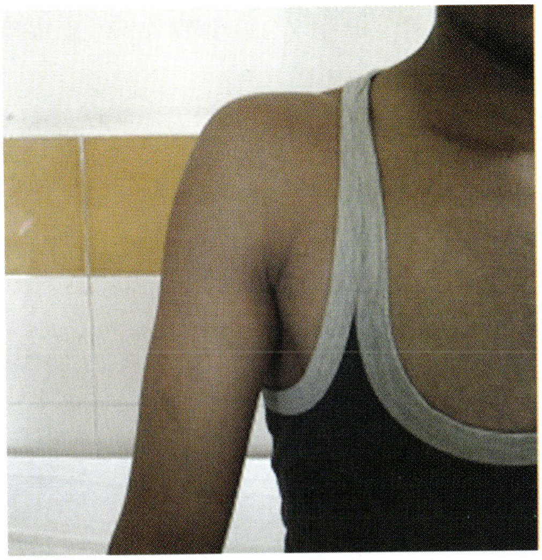

Fig. 9.7(a)

PROCEDURE (Figs. 9.7(a) to (j))

1. Wash and dry the skin, checking for cuts, abrasions or sensitive areas. Shave the upper humerus (arm) and chest area to be taped.
2. Apply skin toughener spray to minimize irritation and improve tape adherence.

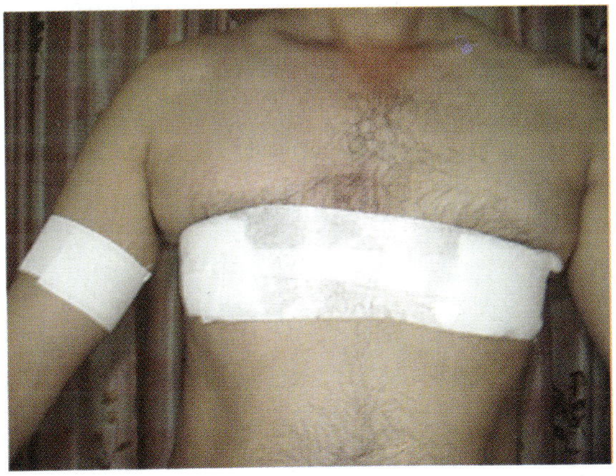

Fig. 9.7(b)

3. Cover the athlete's nipples with gauze, prowrap or felt.
4. Apply two circumferential strips (3 inch) elastic adhesive tape around the thorax with moderate tension.

Tips: Turn athlete's face away and protect the nipple when spraying.

NOTES:

- Check sensation, pulse, temperature and col before starting to tape.
- For female athlete, apply this strip below bre rising up slightly laterally on the injured side.

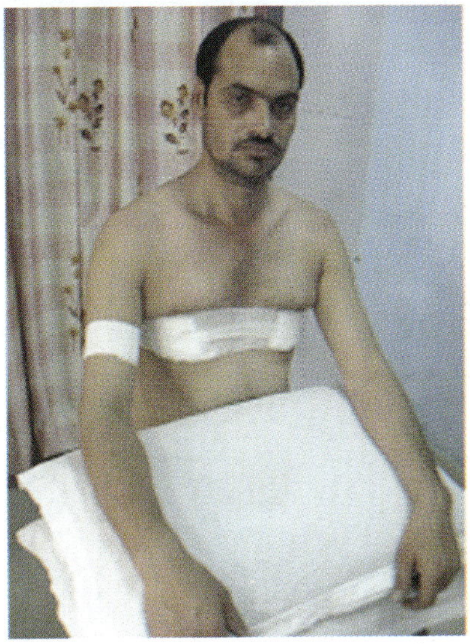

Fig. 9.7(c)

5. Apply two circumferential anchors of 7.5 (3 inch) elastic adhesive tape lightly around the mid humerus (mid upper arm) at the distal end of the deltoid muscle.
6. With moderate tension wrap a circumferential strip of (3 inch) elastic adhesive tape over the thoracic anchor.

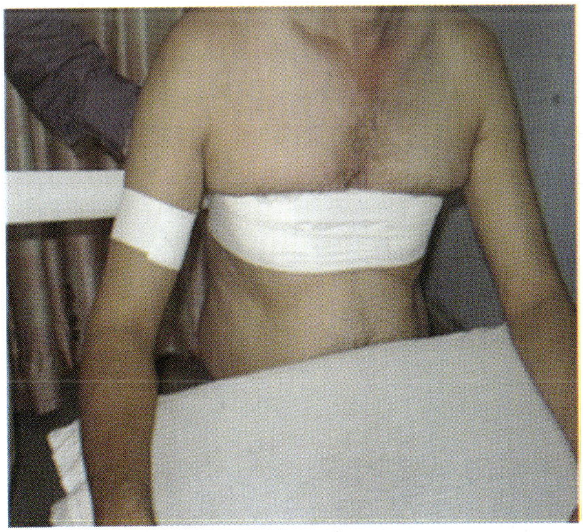

Fig. 9.7(d)

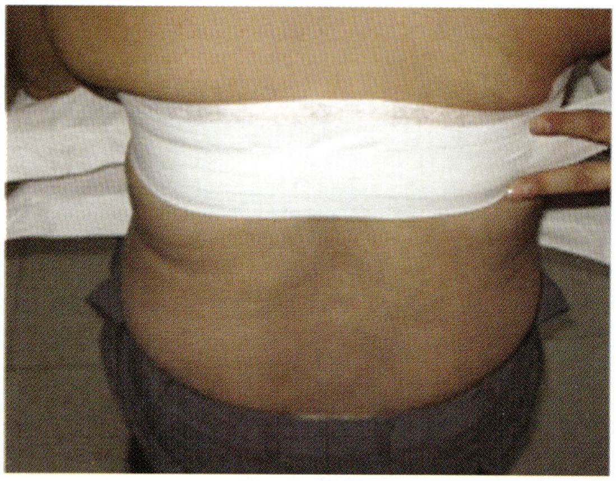

Fig. 9.7(e)

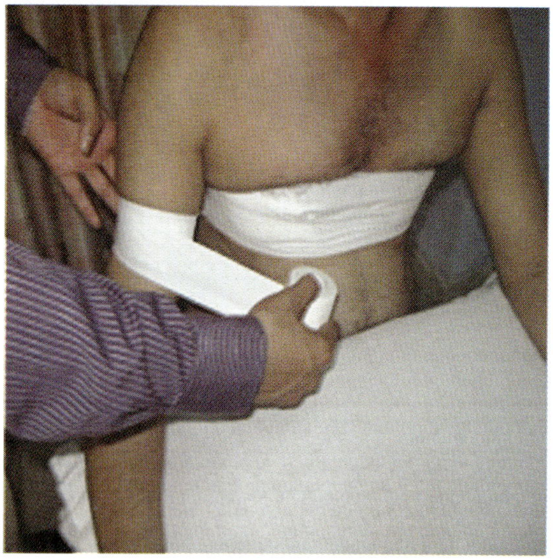

Fig. 9.7(f)

7. Pinch it at the side, form a loop and continue across the anterior chest wall.

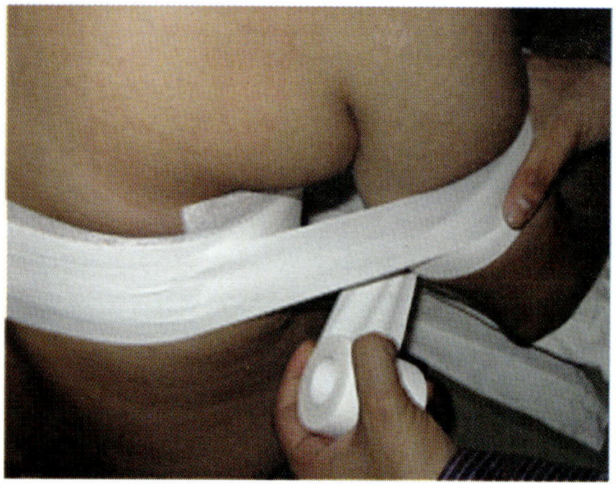

Fig. 9.7(g)

8. Pass a small roll of (1.5 inch) tape through these loops.

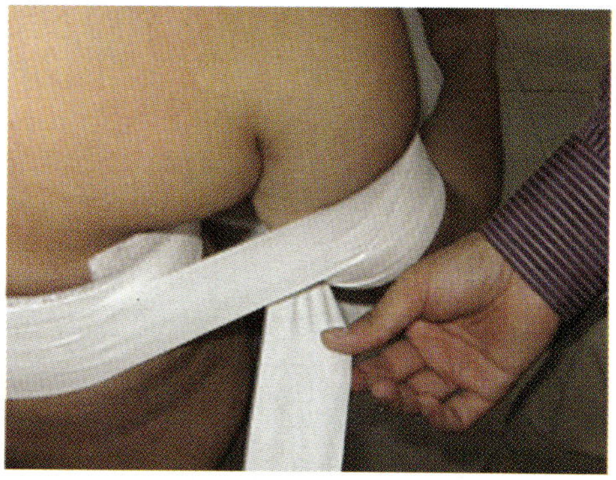

Fig. 9.7(h)

9. Attach them together to form a tether with 1.5 inch white tape.

10. The stability of the shoulder can be cautiously tested at this stage.

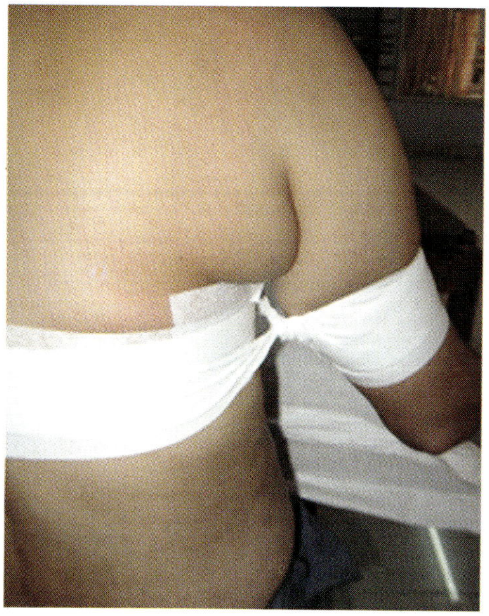

Fig. 9.7(i)

11. Test the degree of restriction:

    a. External rotation must be limited to 30 degree.

    b. Abduction must be limited to 45 degree.

    c. Flexion must be limited.

    d. The athlete must feel secure without any sense of apprehension on stress testing.

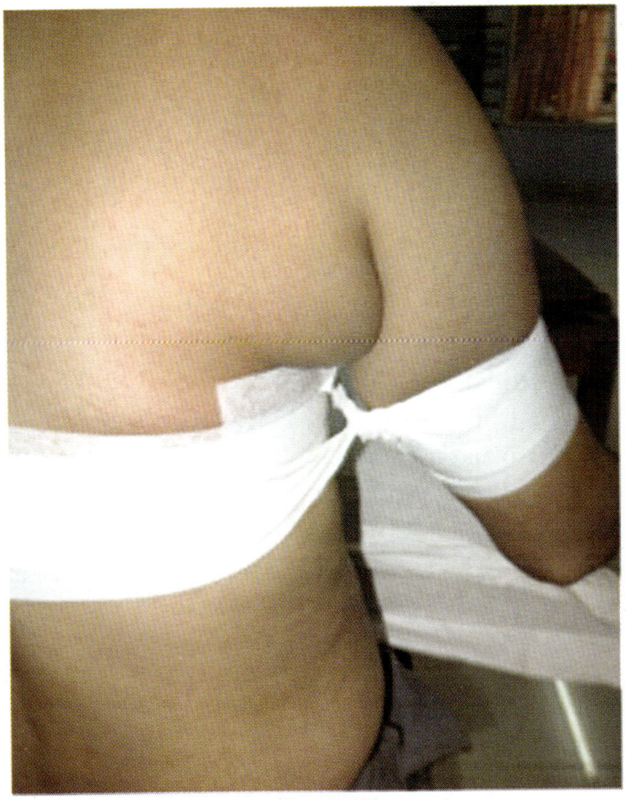

Fig. 9.7(j)

12. Sensation, pulse, strength, temperature and colour must be reassessed to ensure that the taping has not compromised circulation.

10 ELBOW TAPING

At the elbow, the **humero-ulnar** joint (the true elbow joint), is a hinge joint like the knee.

The main purpose and value in taping an elbow is the prevention of full extension of the joint, with or without lateral reinforcement. Because the associated **radio-ulnar (forearm)** joints allow a great degree of pronation and supination (rotation) the overall effectiveness of taping for lateral ligaments is compromised.

LEFT ELBOW FROM THE FRONT

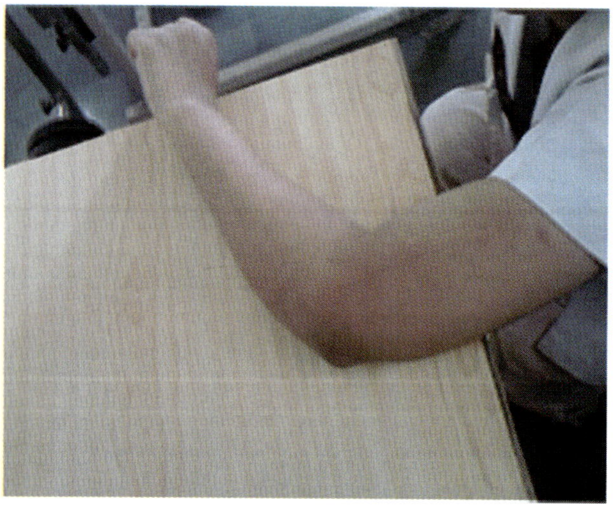

Fig. 10.1

There is an M shaped pattern of superficial vein cephalic and basic veins are joint by a medial cubital vein into which drain two small median forearm veins.

The order of the structures in the cubital fossa forms the lateral to the medial in biceps tendon, brachial artery and median nerve.

X=Crossed Taping

FOREARM FROM THE FRONT

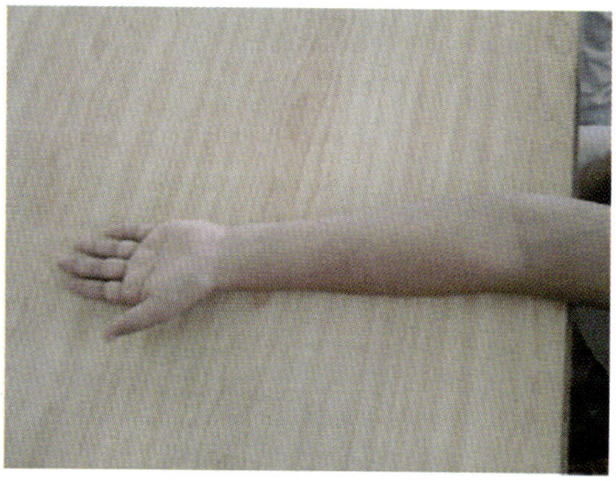

Fig. 10.2

MUSCLES

1. Biceps.
2. Brachioradialis.
3. Pronater teres.
4. Biceps.
5. Flexor carpi radialis.

NERVES

6. Median.

FASCIA

7. Bicipital aponeurosis.

VEINS

8. Basilic.
9. Cephalic vein.
10. Median cephalic vein.

11. Median basilic vein.

12. Median forearm vein.

ARTERIES

13. Brachial.

BONES

14. Medial epicondyle of humerus.

15. Lateral epicondyle of humerus.

With the elbow fully extended, the extensors muscle bulge on the lateral side. In the adjacent hollow can be felt the heal of radius and the capitulum which indicate the line of hum radial part of the elbow joint. The lateral and medial epicondyles of the humerus are palpable on each side. Wrinkled skin lies at the back of the prominent olecranon of the ulna and in this arm the margin of the olecranon bursa is outlined. The most important structure in this region is the ulnar nerve which is palpable as it lies in contact with the humerus behind the medial epicondyles. The posterior border of ulna is subcutaneous throughout its whole length.

- With the elbow extended (straight) the medial and lateral epicondyles of the humerus and the olecranon moves to lower level.
- The subcutaneous position of the ulnar nerve behind the medial epicondyles of the humerus makes it easily palpable: here it can be roll against bone or injured with paraesthesia (tingling sensation) in the distribution of the nerve on the ulnar side of hand.
- The region of the medial epicondyles of the humerus is referred to as the (funny bone).

THE BACK OF FOREARM

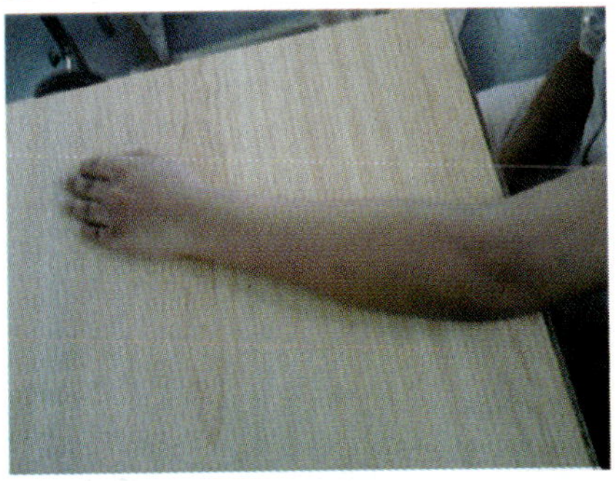

Fig. 10.3

The superficial extensors muscles take a common origin from the lateral epicondyles of the humerus and the supra condoyle ridge. Brachioradialis, the muscle coming from higher up the ridge, has been described with the anterior muscles in view of its flexor role. Extensor carpi radialis longus also comes from the supra condylar ridge below that, extensor carpi radialis brevis arises from the epicondyles.

MUSCLES

1. Brachioradialis.
2. Extensor carpi radialis longus.
3. Extensor carpi radialis brevis.
4. Extensor digitorum.
5. Extensor carpi ulnaris.
6. Triceps.
7. Flexor carpi ulnaris.
8. Anconeus.

BONES

9. Lateral epicondyle of humerus.

10. Medial epicondyle of humerus.

11. Capitulum of humerus.

12. Olecranon of ulna.

13. Posterior border of ulna.

14. Head of radius.

NERVES

15. Ulnar.

BURSA

16. Margin of olecranon bursa.

TAPING FOR ELBOW HYPEREXTENSION SPRAIN

Purpose

- Supports the elbow laterally.

- Limits the last 30 degree of extension and end-range pronation of the forearm.
- Allows the full flexion and almost full supination.

Indications for use

- Acute, sub-acute or chronic hyperextension sprains of the elbow.
- Posterior impingement syndrome.
- Medial sprains of the elbow, supported by reinforcing the medial X strips.
- Lateral sprains of the elbow, supported by reinforcing the lateral X strips.
- Combination of ligament sprains.
- Chronic instability following fracture, dislocation of the elbow.

NOTES:
- Ensure a proper diagnosis by a sports physiotherapist.
- X-rays should be taken to rule out possibility fracture.
- Pain or laxity on lateral stress testing with the elbow at 15 degree flexion, will indicate the need for added medial or lateral support.
- Easily irritated structures include the biceps tendon, soft in elbow crease and the ulnar nerve or funny bone, found posterio-mediality in the groove.
- If forearm anchor is too tight, circulation of the forearm will be constricted.

MATERIALS

- Razor.
- Skin toughener spray.
- Prowrap.
- (2 inch) elastic adhesive tape.
- (3 inch) elastic adhesive tape.
- (1.5 inch)white non-elastic adhesive tape.
- (3 inch) elastic wrap bandage.

TERMINOLOGY

- Sprain of medial or lateral collateral ligaments.
- Tearing of anterior joint capsule.

ETIOLOGY

- Fall on outstretched hand.
- Forced hyperextension of the elbow (anterior capsule with/without medial and /or lateral ligament sprain).
- Forced valgus (inward) stress causes damage to the medial collateral ligament (more vulnerable and more common).
- Forced varus (outward) stress causes damage to the damage to the medial collateral ligament.
- Chronic medial sprains are common in pitchers and javelin throwers.

SYMPTOMS

- Pain on anterior capsule–medial and/or lateral joint line–implies localized injury site.
- Swelling.
- Active movement testing: Pain on end-range extension.
- Resistance testing: Neutral position.
  a. No significant pain on moderate resistance.
  b. Pain on flexion if biceps simultaneously injured.
- Stress testing: Varying degrees of pain and laxity on stress testing (done at 15 degree flexion) amount of laxity indicates degree of injury.

NOTE: Any suspicion of deformity requires immediate medical attention and X-ray.

TREATMENT

Early

- R.I.C.E.S.
- Sling.
- Therapeutic modalities.

Later

Continued physiotherapy including:

- Therapeutic modalities.
- Taping for limited activity: **For elbow hyperextension taping.**

- Progressive resistance rehabilitation program for humero-ulnar as well as radio-ulnar joints.
- Gradual return to activities with taped support.

SEQUELAE

- Chronic instability.
- Ulnar nerve paraesthesia.
- Adhesions causing reduced range of motion.
- Arthritic changes.
- Calcification of ligaments.

POSITIONING

Sitting, with the elbow held in 40 degree flexion. The forearm should be in a neutral position between pronation and supination with the hand in functional position.

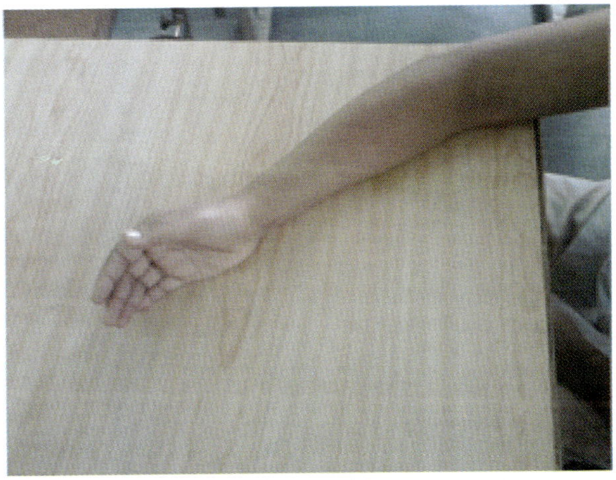

Fig. 10.4(a)

PROCEDURE (Figs. 10.4(a) to (l))

1. Wash the skin, dry, and check for cuts, abrasions or sensitive areas.
2. Spray the elbow up to and including the shaved bands of skin with skin toughener.

NOTE: Sensation, pulse, temperature and colour of hand must be cheeked prior to taping.

3. Apply prowrap from the proximal (upper) one-third of the forearm to the distal (lower) one-third of the humerus.

NOTE: Padding and lubricant may be applied on the anterior aspect of the elbow to protect the biceps tendon and the soft skin when returning to sports with significant repetitive elbow motion.

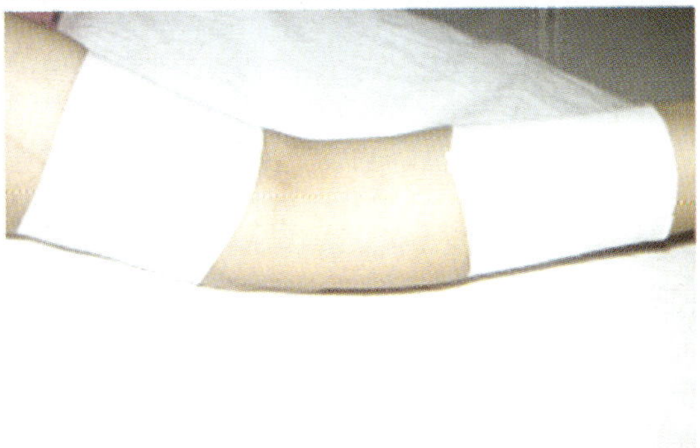

Fig. 10.4(b)

4. Apply 2 circumferential anchors of (2 inch) elastic adhesive tape with minimal tension to the mid-humerus half-covering the prowrap and half-covering the skin directly.

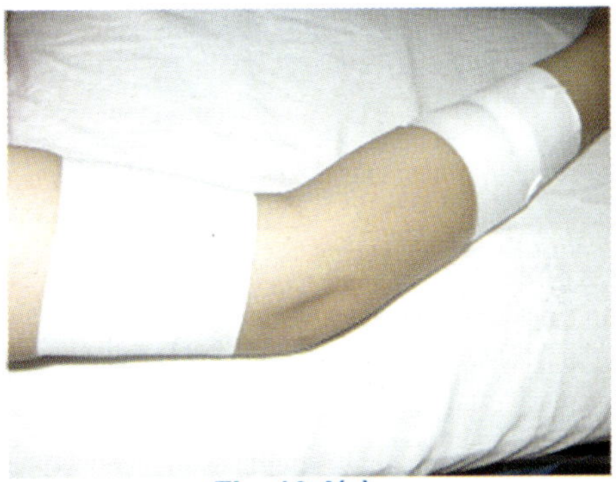

Fig. 10.4(c)

5. Repeat 2 similar anchors mid to lower forearm.

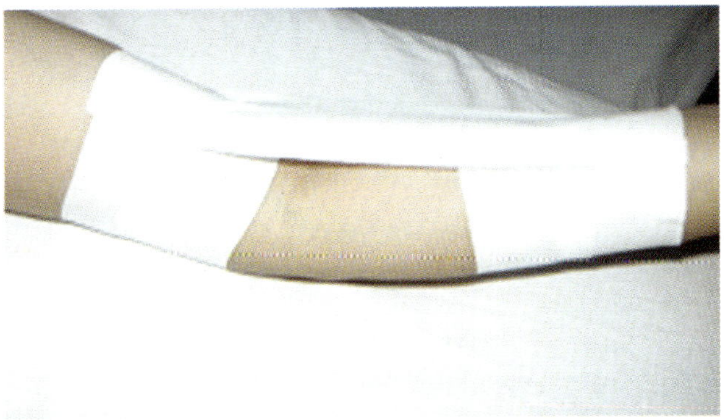

Fig. 10.4(d)

6. To form a check-rein place the elbow in 45 degree of flexion and apply a vertical strip of (2 inch) elastic adhesive tape from the lower anchor with tension to the upper anchor, directly over the anterior aspect of the elbow joint.

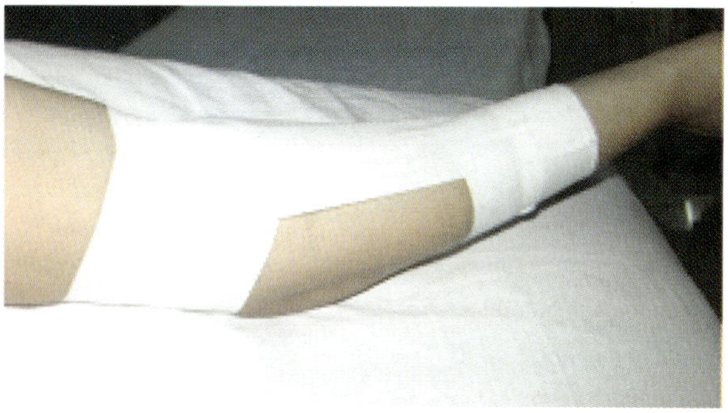

Fig. 10.4(e)

7. Repeat this strip overlapped by ½ the tape width more laterally.

Tips: Be certain to apply these strips with enough tension to block the last 30 degree of extension when elbow is fully stretched.

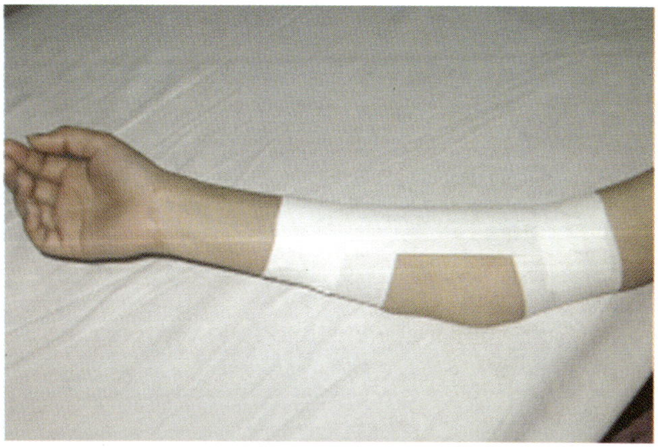

Fig. 10.4(f)

8. Anchor these strips at both ends.

Tips: Remember to keep the hand in a functional position.

9. For medial stability, hold the elbow bent at 35 degree of flexion, and applies a vertical strip (1.5 inch) white tape from the distal anchor to the upper anchor with strong tension.

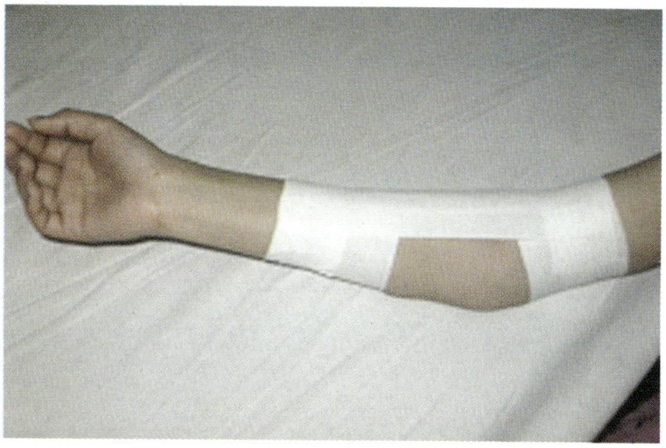

Fig. 10.4(g)

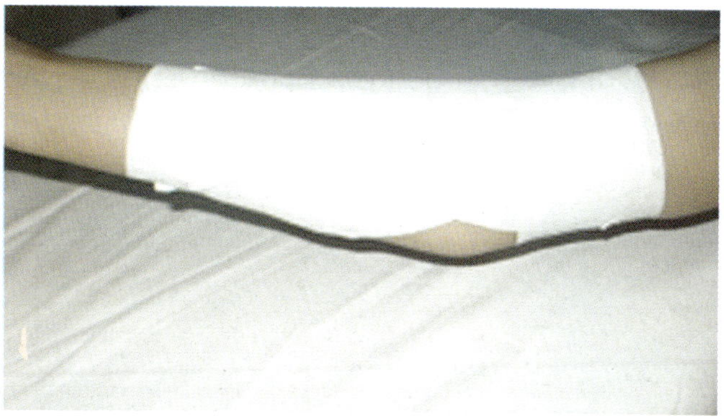

Fig. 10.4(h)

10. Apply a several strip to form an X across the medial joint line of the elbow also with strong tension.

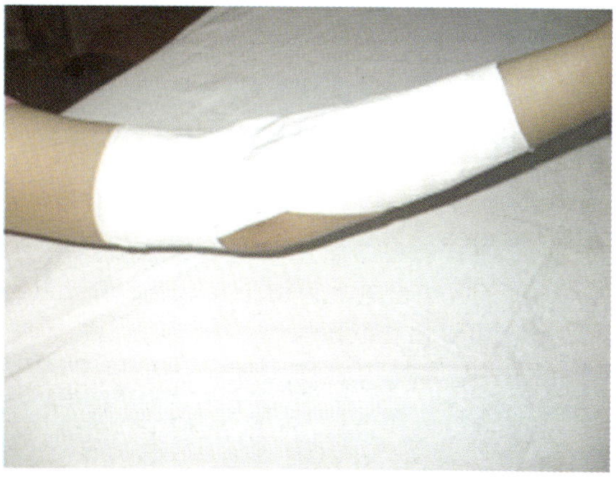

Fig. 10.4(i)

11. Repeat the white tape X on the lateral aspect to cross at the lateral joint line.

NOTE: For lateral sprains ensure a more valgus (outwardly bent) position and apply a second white X on the lateral side with great tension.

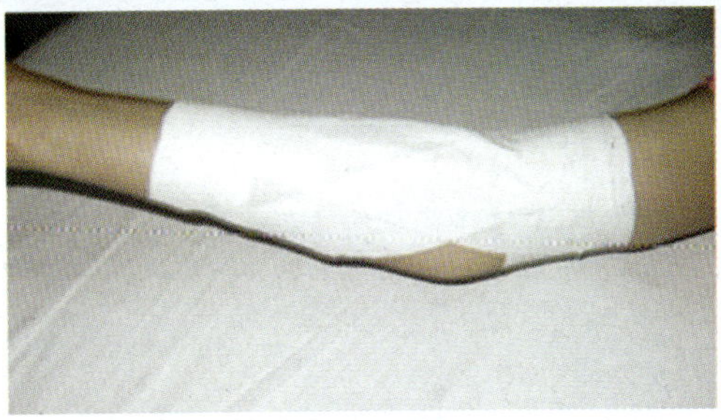

Fig. 10.4(j)

12. Apply two anchors distally and proximally using (3 inch) elastic adhesive tape.

NOTE: In closing up, a space is left at the anterior elbow, to avoid undue irritation to he sensitive underlying structures.

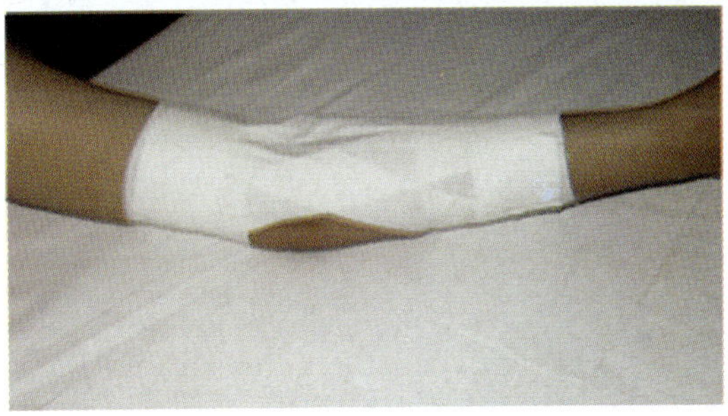

Fig. 10.4(k)

13. Anterior view of finishing taping.

NOTE: Hand sensation, pulse, temperature and colour must be reassessed to ensure that taping has not compromised circulation.

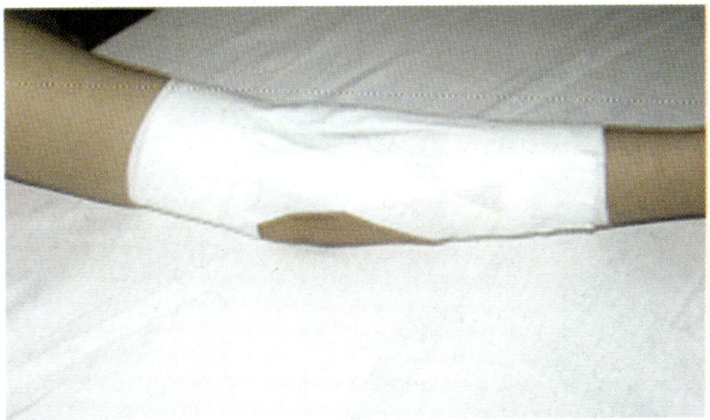

Fig. 10.4(l)

14. Test the degree of restriction:
    a. Extension should be limited by 30 degree or more.
    b. There should be no pain on passive extension or lateral stress testing.

Tips: Wrap the tape job with a 7.5 cm (3 inch) tensor bandage for 10 minutes to ensure good adherence.

11 WRIST AND HAND TAPING

WRIST AND HAND

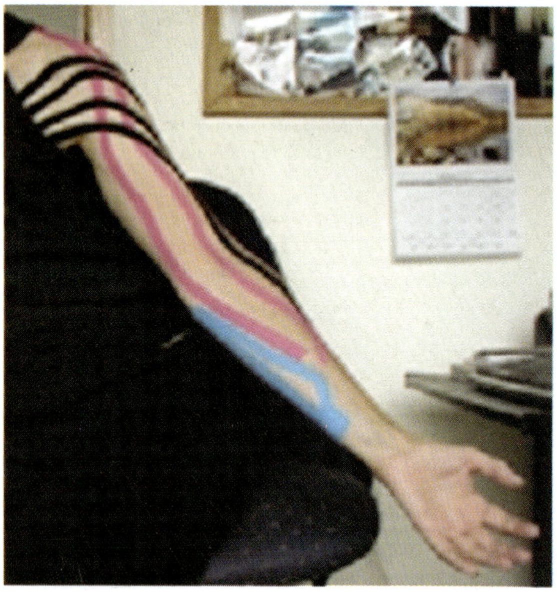

Fig. 11.1

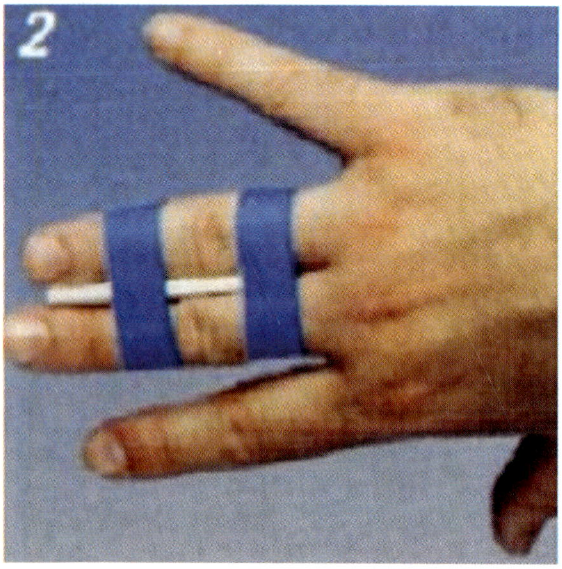

Fig. 11.2

X=Crossed Taping

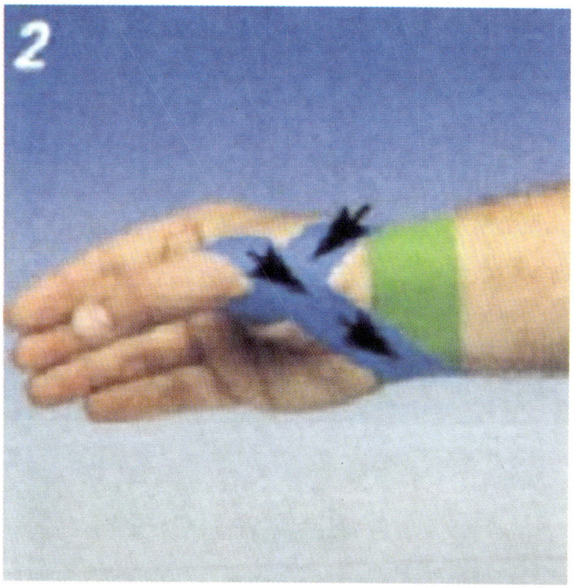

Fig. 11.3

The **wrist** is liable osteo-ligamentous complex forming a connecting link between the forearm and the hand. Multidirectional mobility results from the numerous multi-articular carpal bones which, along with the radio-ulnar joints, allow the hand to be positioned functionally at any angle. Stability is derived from the complex array of ligaments often injure when falling on an outstretched hand. Vascular supply to the carpal bones is often compromised with ligamentous damage.

The **hand,** while being the most active and intricate joint complex in the body, is the least protected. Constructed as a series of complex, delicately balanced joints, it offers manipulating ability, dexterity and precision. This highly sensitive structure used to hold, hit, catch and manipulate, is particularly vulnerable to trauma when subjected to repetitive stresses or the impact of falls.

Providing adequate support while still maintaining functional movement is the prime consideration when taping the hand and/or wrist.

SURFACE MARKINGS

The surface markings of various structures within the wrist and hand are indicated, not all of them are palpable e.g. the superficial and deep palm.

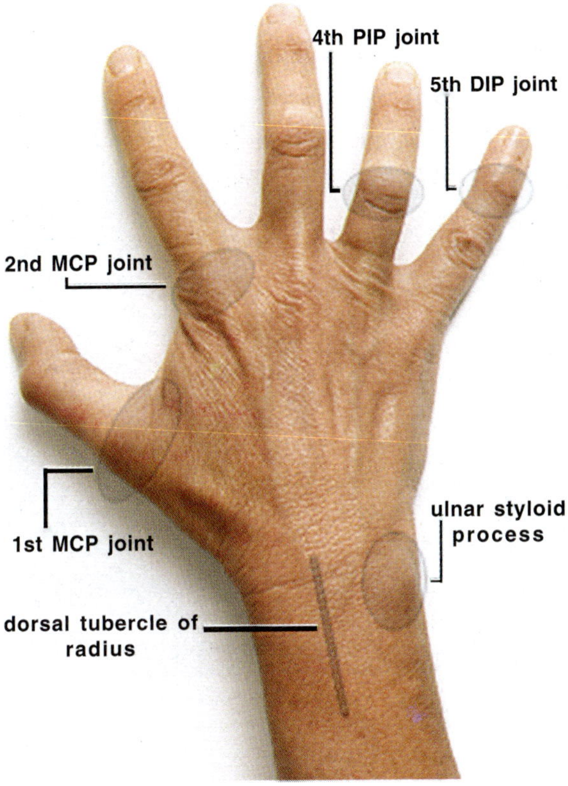

Fig. 11.4

CREASES

1. Longitudinal.
2. Proximal transverse.
3. Distal transverse.
4. Distal wrist.
5. Middle wrist.
6. Proximal wrist.

ARCHES

7. Superficial palmar.
8. Deep palmar.

MUSCLES

9. Abductor digiti minimi.
10. Flexor digiti minimi.
11. Palmaris brevis.
12. Abductor pollicis.
13. Flexor pollicis brevis.
14. Thenor eminence.
15. Adductor pollicis.

ARTERIS

16. Ulnar and radial.

TENDONS

17. Flexor carpi ulnaris.
18. Palmaris longus brevis.
19. Flexor carpi radialis.

BONES

20. Head of metacarpal.
21. Hook of hamate.
22. Pisiform.

Surface anatomy: Dorsum and palmar of the hand.

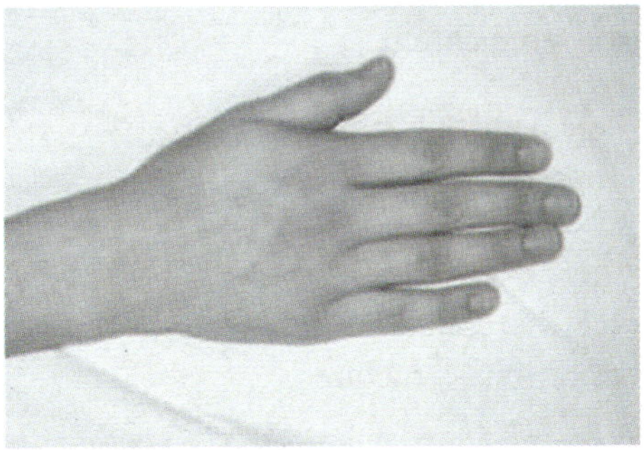

Fig. 11.5

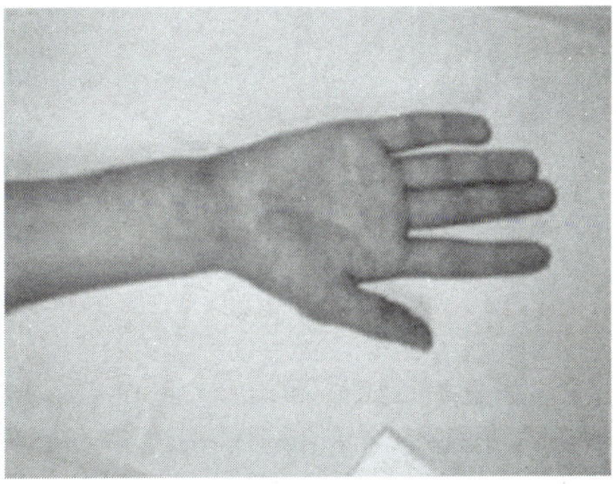

Fig. 11.6

TENDONS

1. Extensor digiti minimi.
2. Extensor digitorum.
3. Extensor indices.
4. Extensor carpi radialis longus.
5. Extensor pollicis longus.
6. Extensor pollicis brevis.
7. Abductor pollicis longus.

MUSCLES

8. First dorsal interosseus.

BONES

9. Anatomical snuff box over scaphoid.
10. Styloid process of radius.
11. Head of ulna.

VEINS

12. Cephalic.

RETINACULUM

13. Extensor retinaculum.

WRIST HYPEREXTENSION SPRAIN TAPING

Purpose

- Reinforce the collateral ligaments of the wrist and the anterior joint structures.
- Restricts extension and limits the last degrees of radial and ulnar deviation (sideways movement).
- Permits functional use of the hand.

Indications for use

- Palmar radio-carpal ligament (wrist hyperextension) sprains.
- For dorsal radio-carpal ligament (wrist hyper flexion) sprains: Apply the check rein dorsally (back of wrist) and add restraining Xs to the dorsal aspect of the wrist thus limiting end-range flexion.
- For radial collateral ligament sprains: Reinforce the lateral X and add a lateral palmar X to prevent ulnar deviation.
- For ulnar collateral ligament sprain: reinforce the medial X and add a medial palmar X to prevent radial deviation.
- Diffuse pain in the wrist due to repeated compression, or jamming the wrist.
- Wrist pain post immobilization.

NOTES:

- Ensure that a proper diagnosis has been made to rule out fractures–particularly if the injury was caused by a fall on the outstretched hand (the scaphoid bone [first carpal bone at the base of the thumb]is the most commonly fractured).
- Clarify the mechanism of injury, whether it was hyperextension that occurred.
- The use of skin toughener or quick dry adhesive spray is essential for adherence of taping, especially in rainy or hot conditions when hands, wrists and forearms tend to become quite damp.

MATERIALS

- Razor.
- Skin toughener spray.
- Prowrap.
- 3.8 cm (1.5 inch) white tape.

TERMINOLOGY

- Partial or complete tearing of anterior wrist capsule.
- Partial or complete tearing of radial and/or ulnar collateral ligaments.

ETIOLOGY

- Fall on outstretched hand.
- Forced hyperextension during a tackle with an opponent.
- Overloaded weight lifting.

SYMPTOMS

- Pain over anterior joint capsule and ligaments.
- Decreased range of motion.
- Swelling.
- Active movement testing: Pain on end range extension.
- Passive movement testing:
  a. Pain on extension.
  b. Pain possible on end-range flexion resulting from compression of injured tissues.
- Resistance testing (neutral position): No significant pain with moderate resistance; pain possible on flexion if flexors also involved.
- Stress testing: Varying degrees of pain and laxity.

NOTE: If wrist is unstable when testing ligaments, X-rays must be taken to rule out the possibility of fracture.

TREATMENT

Early

- R.I.C.E.S.
- Initially: Elastic tensor compression and sling support with careful attention to circulation for the first 48 hours.
- Therapeutic modalities, contrast baths.

Later

Continued physiotherapy including:

- Therapeutic modalities.
- Flexibility exercises.
- Strengthening (isometric initially).
- Total rehabilitation program for mobility, flexibility, strengthening and dexterity.
- Taping for gradual return to pain-free functional act.

NOTE: Sprain that does not respond well to treatment should be reassessed by a hand specialist. Pain and clicking on ulnar side may imply damage to the triangular fibro-cartilage (meniscus).Persistent pain on the radial side may indicate a necrosis or missed fracture of the scaphoid (circulation of the carpal bones often compromised with wrist sprains.

SEQUELAE

- Tenosynovitis.
- Weakness.
- Chronic pain.
- Instability.
- Degenerative joint changes.
- Stubborn cases may suggest an associated meniscal tear and require some form of splitting for dynamic activity.

POSITIONING

Sitting with the wrist in a neutral position held in slight extension (approximately 20 degree).

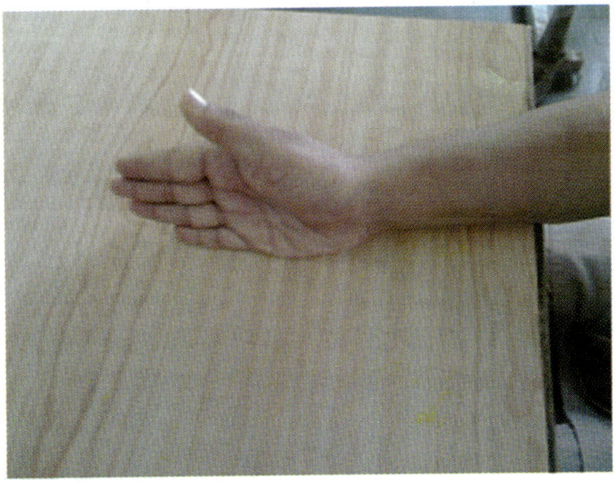

Fig. 11.7(a)

PROCEDURE (Figs. 11.7(a) to (h))

1. Wash, dry and shave, the forearm, if hairy. Check for cuts, abrasions and sensitive skin.
2. Spray the area to be taped.

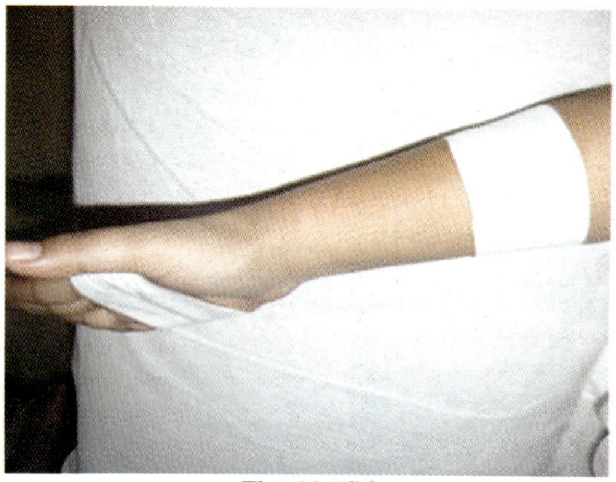

Fig. 11.7(b)

3. Apply 2 circumferential anchors of (1.5 inch) white tape around mid-forearm at musculo-tendinous junction, following the soft tissue contours.

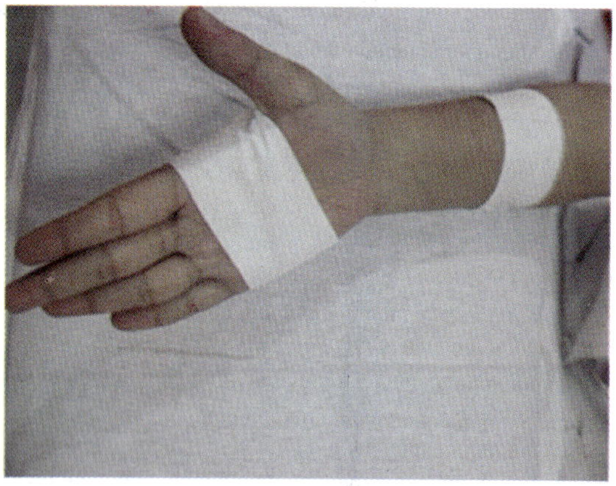

Fig. 11.7(c)

4. Apply a circumferential anchor of white tape around the distal metacarpals (palm of hand).

Tips: Ensure that these anchors do not unduly restrict splaying of the metacarpals.

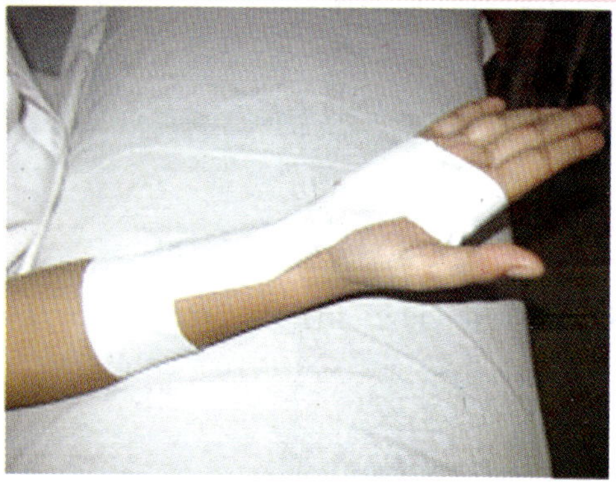

Fig. 11.7(d)

5. Hold the wrist at 0 degree extension and apply a check-rein (restraining strip) from the anterior aspect of the distal anchor to the proximal, with strong tension, passing across the anterior joint line.

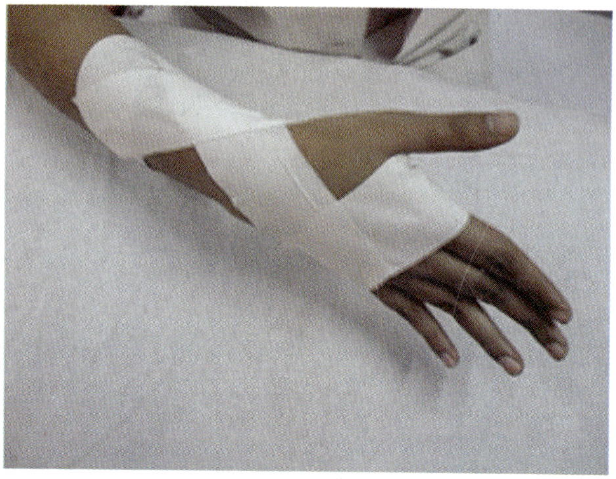

Fig. 11.7(e)

6. Start the medial X from the anterior aspect of the distal anchor to the posterior-medial aspect of the proximal anchor.
7. Finish the X with a strip from the posterior-medial aspect of the distal anchor to the proximal anchor anteriorly with firm tension.

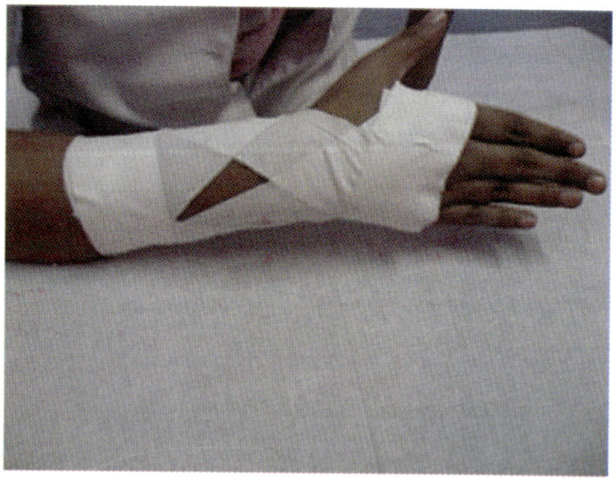

Fig. 11.7(f)

8. Begin a lateral X with a strip from the posterior aspect of the distal anchor pulling with tension to the anterior aspect of the proximal anchor.
9. Finish this X with a strip from the anterior aspect of the distal anchor to the lateral aspect of the proximal anchor.

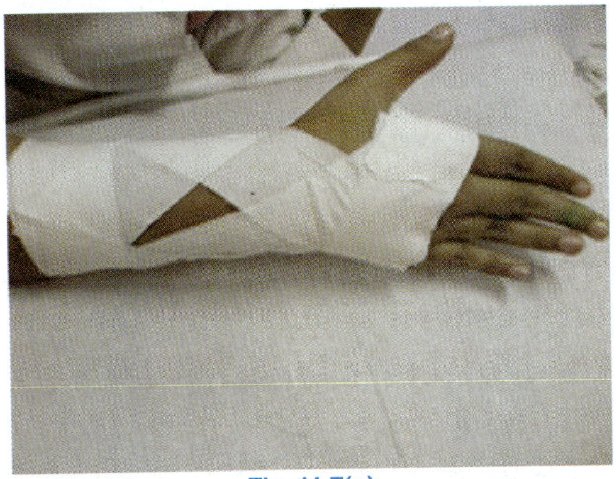

Fig. 11.7(g)

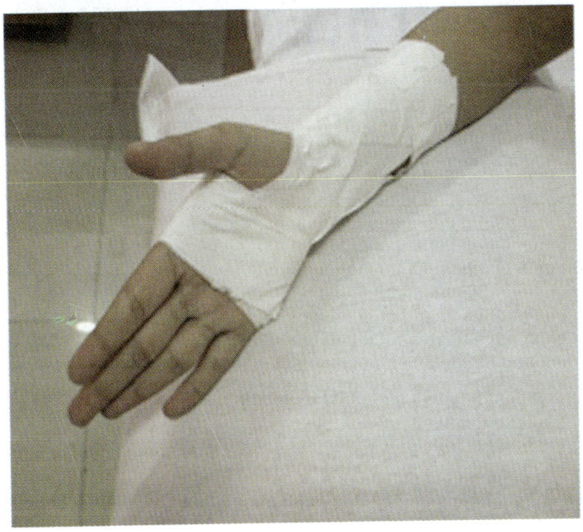

Fig. 11.7(h)

10. Re-anchor these supporting X both distally and proximally.
11. Test the degree of restriction: Extension should be limited to 30 degree or less. There must be no pain on passive extension at the wrist.

NOTE: Check figure colour and sensation or signs of compromised circulation.

THUMB SPRAIN TAPING

Purpose

- Supports the collateral ligaments of the first metacarpal phalange joint.
- Prevents the last degrees of extension, limits abduction.
- Allows some flexion.
- Does not compromise wrist and hand function.

Indications for use

- Metacarpo-phalangeal joint (MCPJ) sprain (ulnar ligament).
- Carp metacarpal joint (CMCJ) sprain (ulnar aspect); reinforce the diagonal anchor.
- Skiers thumb, gamekeepers thumb.
- Post-immobilization tenderness.
- Post-surgery of 3rd degree repair.

NOTES:
- If a 3rd degree sprain be suspected (greater than 35 degree of adduction) a hand surgeon should be seen as early as possible.
- X-ray will rule out the possibility of an avulsion fracture.
- Thoroughly inspect the hand of cuts , abrasions and any other possible sources of infection.
- Watch carefully for signs of restricted circulation particularly during the first 48 hours post-injury when swelling tends to be greatest.
- Restricted circulation, apart, from causing discomfort, can be particularly dangerous in below-freezing weather (increased risk of frost bite).
- Hand and thumb size will dictate the width of tape required.

TERMINOLOGY

- Partial or complete tearing of ulnar collateral ligament: The first MCPJ (Metacarpo-phalangeal joint); degree of severity 1st-3rd.
- **"Game-keepers thumb"**.
- **"Skiers thumb"**.

ETIOLOGY

- Forced extension and/or abduction of the metacarpo-phalangeal joint.

- A fall on an outstretched hand.
- Common in skiing.

SYMPTOMS

- Tenderness over medial aspect of metacarpo-phalangeal joint (base of thumb in the web space).
- Local swelling and/or discolouration.
- Active movement testing: Pain on end-range extension.
- Passive movement testing: Pain on extension plus abduction.
- Resistance testing (Neutral position): No significant pain on moderate resistance.
- Stress testing: More than 35 degree lateral of laxity in both flexion and extension indicates a complete rupture or an avulsion fracture.

TREATMENT

Early

- R.I.C.E.S.
- Therapeutic modalities; contrast bath.
- Range of motion (ROM) exercises.
- Taping: For thumb sprain taping.

> **NOTE:** 3rd degree and severe 2nd degree require spica splint, casting or surgery with at least 3 weeks of immobilization.

LATER

Continued physiotherapy including:

- Therapeutic modalities.
- Joint mobilizations if post-immobilization.
- Strengthening (isometric at first).
- Gradual return to pain-free functional activities with taped support.
- Complete rehabilitation program including range of motion, flexibility, strengthening and dexterity.

SEQUELAE

- Chronic instability with severe dysfunction.
- Weakness of grip.
- Tenosynovitis.
- Degenerative changes of metacarpal-phalangeal joint.

POSITIONING

Hand in supination with hand resting on a table in neutral position.

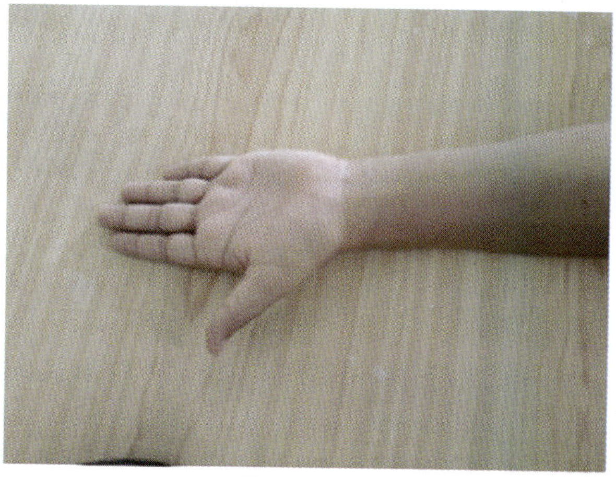

Fig. 11.8(a)

PROCEDURE (Figs. 11.8(a) to (j))

1. Wash, dry and spray the area to be taped.
2. Apply two circumferential strips of (1.5 inch) white tape around the wrist using light tension.

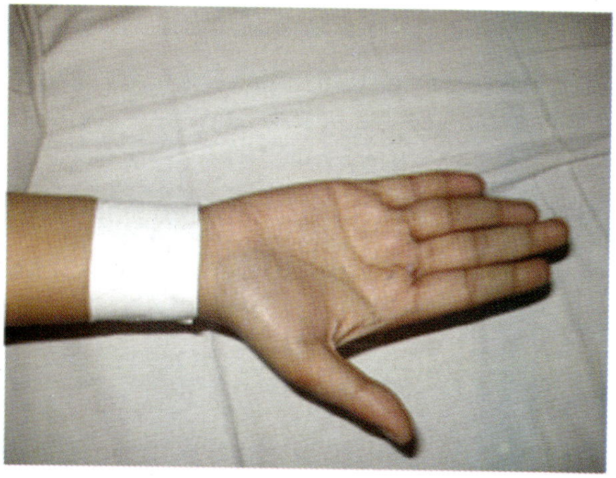

Fig. 11.8(b)

3. Apply the distal anchor.

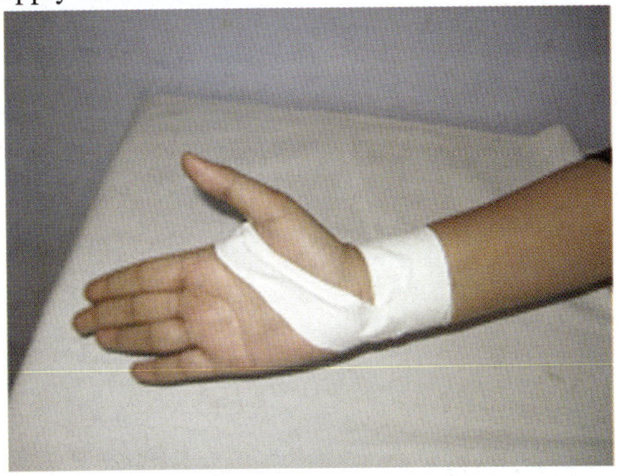

Fig. 11.8(c)

4. Using (1.5 in.) white tape. Start from the posterior side of the proximal anchor, wrap around the wrist, and pull up and across the dorsum of the hand.

   a. Cross from posterior to anterior between the thumb and index finger.

   b. Pinch the tape as it passes through the web space, to narrow the tape and to avoid irritating the soft skin at this site.

Tips: Be careful not to apply any pressure through the web space.

   c. Continue diagonally across the palmar aspect of the hand and fix the strip medially on the proximal anchor.

5. Apply the thumb anchor lightly, placing the strip circumferentially around the proximal phalanx following its contours.

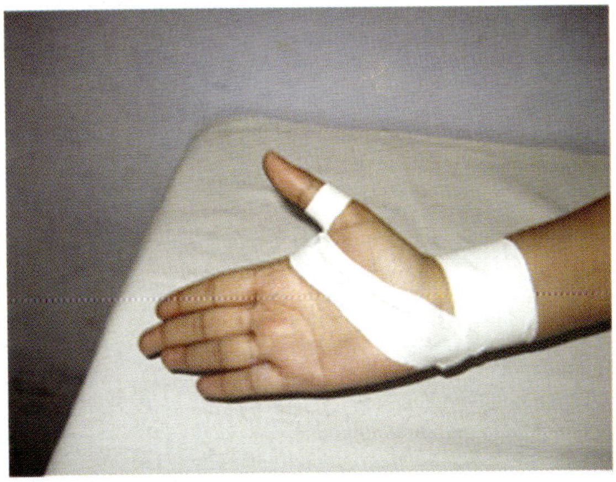

Fig. 11.8(d)

6. Apply an incomplete Figure 8 strip of (0.5 inch) white tape by pulling gently around the thumb crossing the strips and pulling equally with both hands medially, adducting the thumb before adhereing both ends of this strip to the anchor.

7. The anterior end is applied to the palmar anchor, and the posterior end is applied to the dorsal anchor with firm pressure.

Tips: Be careful not to apply strong pressure circumferentially around the thumb during application of tape.

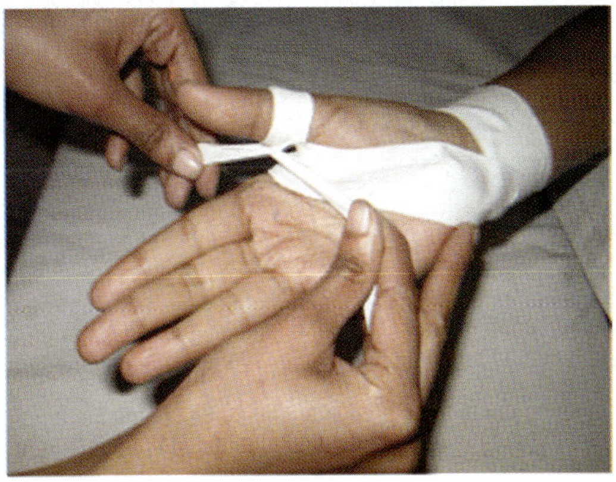

Fig. 11.8(e)

8. a. Apply another half–Figure 8 proximally overlapping by 2/3 the width of the tape on the thumb anchor.

   b. Allow the strip ends fan out slightly as they reach the anchor.

9. Continue repeating the half–Figure 8s overlapping by ½ to 2/3 the width of the tape, moving proximally down the thumb.

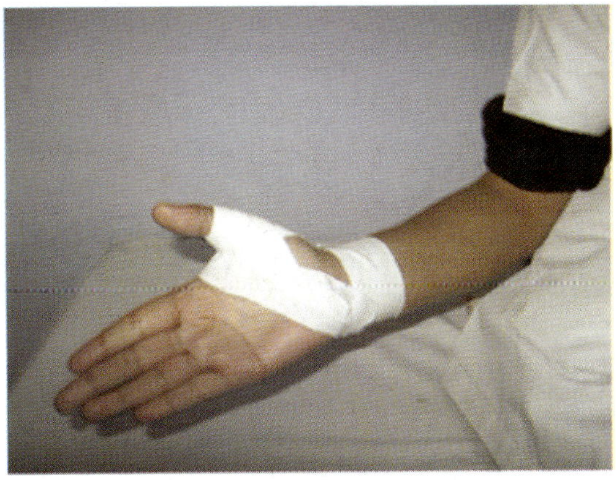

Fig. 11.8(f)

10. Re-anchor the ends of the incomplete Figure 8s with another diagonal anchor.

Tips: Be careful not to apply strong pressure through the web space.

A Figure 8 check-rein can be applied between the thumb and first finger to further restrict abduction.

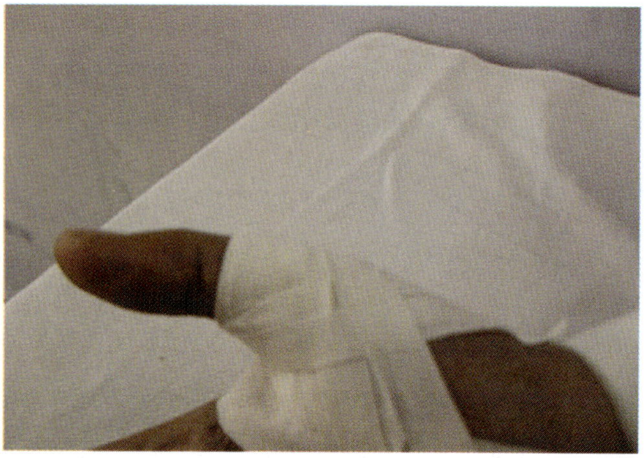

Fig. 11.8(g)

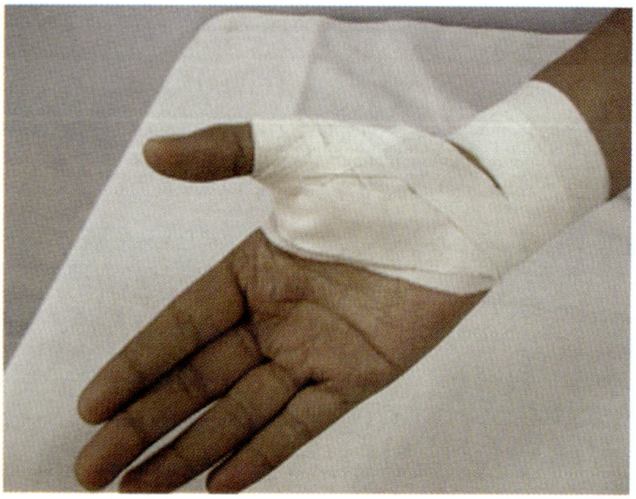

Fig. 11.8(h)

11. Apply circumferential strips of 3.8 cm (1.5 inch) white tape around the wrist covering the diagonal anchor and any remaining tape ends.

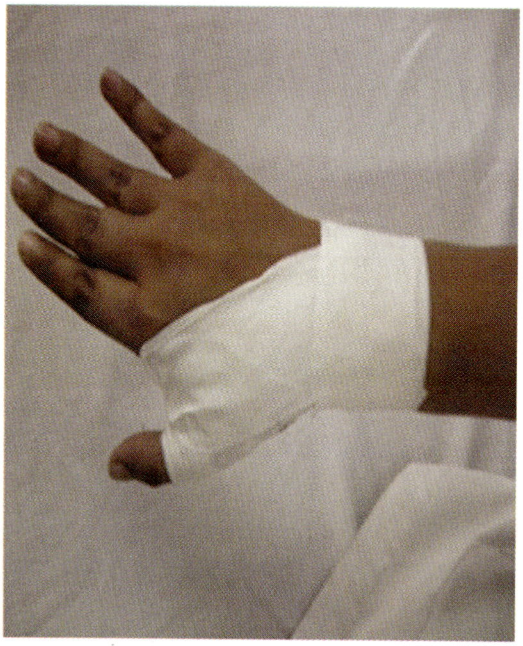

Fig. 11.8(i)

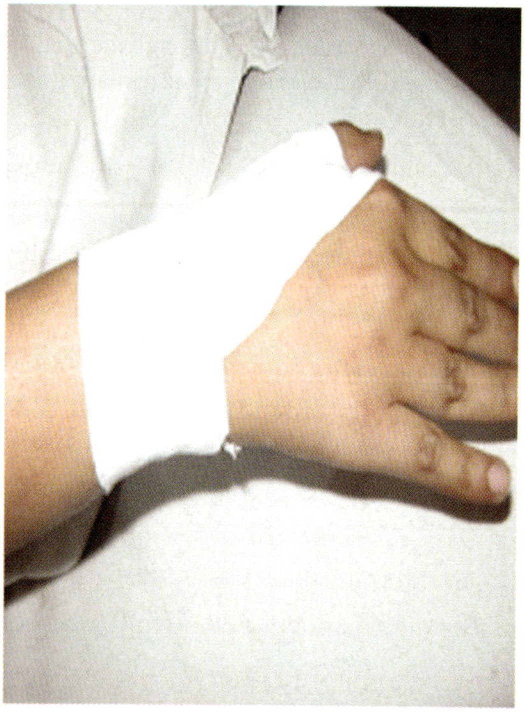

Fig. 11.8(j)

NOTE: Check thumb colour and sensation for signs of compromised circulation restrict abduction.

12. Check functional position of the hand and test the degree of restriction: Extension and abduction must be limited by 20 or more. There should be no pain on passive movements of the thumb particularly extension and abduction must be limited by 20 degree or more. There should be no pain on passive movements of the thumb particularly extension and abduction.

FINGER SPRAIN TAPING

Purpose

- Supports the palmar and collateral ligaments of the finger.
- Prevents full extension.
- Allows full flexion.

Indications for uses

- Palmar ligament sprain (hyperextension) of the finger.
- Post-immobilization painful stiffness of the finger.
- **Jammed** or **stabbed finger.**
- Medial collateral ligament (MCL) sprain of the finger: Reinforce medial X.
- Lateral collateral ligament (LCL) sprain of the finger: Reinforce lateral X.

NOTES:

- Never allow the athlete to continue playing (even when taped).if a serious injury is suspected.
- Ensure a correct diagnosis by a sports physiotherapist (fracture and dislocations are often misdiagnosed and mistreated).
- Localize the exact site of the injury: Which aspect of which joint of which finger, and re-test for pain through range during and after the tape job is completed.
- Taping the injured finger to its neighbour (buddy taping) further protects the injured ligaments while allowing function and movement.
- If the athlete needs to use the injured hand to handle a ball during a game, ("buddy tape") the fingers slightly apart to allow better control of the ball.

MATERIALS

- Razor.
- Skin toughener spray.
- (0.5 inch) white tape.

TERMINOLOGY

- Partial or complete rupture of palmar ligament (anterior capsule), medial collateral (ulnar) ligament or lateral collateral (radial) ligaments: degree of severity: 1st-3rd.
- **"Stoved Finger".**
- **"Jammed Finger".**

ETIOLOGY

- Telescoping below: Direct compressive force on the tip of finger (i.e. jamming it against a ball as in basketball or volleyball).
- Torsional stresses.
- Sideways stress to a finger: May catch on clothing, equipment or terrain.
- Hyperextension of finger.
- Contusion of ligaments.

SYMPTOMS

- Pain over site of injury.
- Swelling and discolouration.
- Local tenderness.
- Active movement testing: Pain on end-range extension and/or flexion (pinching the injured capsule).
- Passive movement testing: Pain on end range extension and/or possibly on flexion.
- Resistance testing: (Neutral position): No significant pain on moderate resistance.
- Stress testing:
  a. Pain with or without laxity on lateral stress testing in 1st and 2nd degree sprains.
  b. Instability with 3rd degree sprains (often with less pain).

TREATMENT

Early

- R.I.C.E.S.
- Initial taping: loose "**Buddy Taping".**
- Therapeutic modalities; contrast baths.
- Range of motion exercises.

NOTE : 3rd degree and severe 2nd degree sprains usually require splinting with at least one week of complete immobilization between treatments and range of motion (ROM) exercises, followed by eight weeks of taped support.

Later

Continued physiotherapy including:

- Therapeutic modalities.
- Mobilizations.
- Flexibility.
- Strengthening exercises for all hand musculature.
- Taping for gradual return to pain-free functional activities for thumb sprain taping.
- Progressive exercises for range of motion strength and dexterity.

SEQUEQLAE

- Persistent laxity (instability).
- Chronic sprain re-injury.
- Deformity.
- Stiffness.
- Degenerative joint changes.

POSITIONING (Figs. 11.9(a) to (j)

Sitting with the elbow supported on a table and the fingers placed in a neutral, functional position.

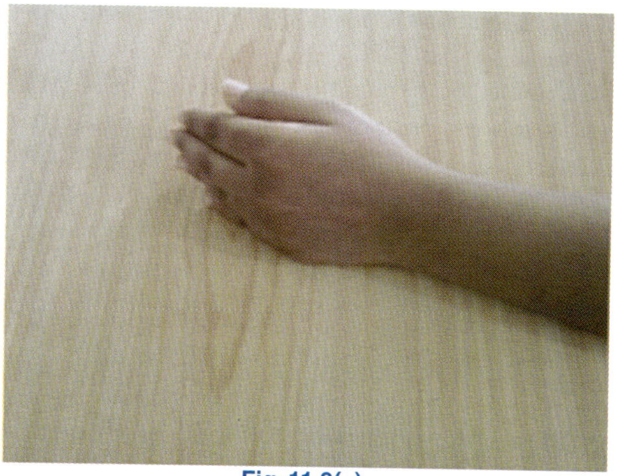

Fig. 11.9(a)

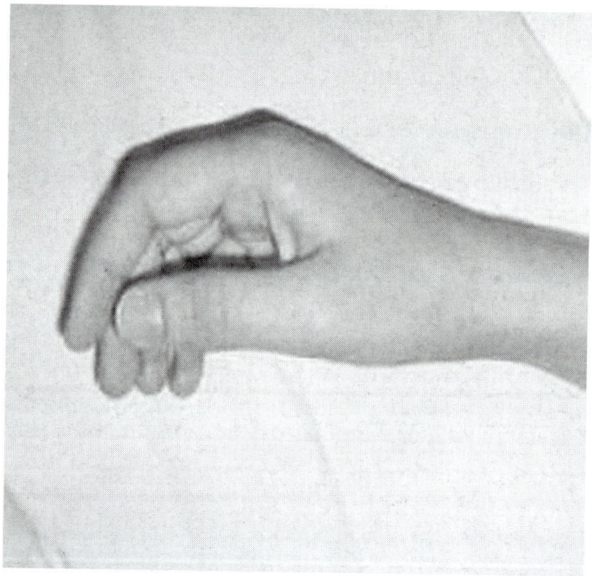

Fig. 11.9(b)

PROCEDURE

1. Wash and dry finger, watching for cuts or abrasions.
2. Spray the area with skin toughener or adhesive spray.

Tips : A cotton-tip applicator can be used to minimize the adherence of non-affected digits.

3. Gently apply two circumferential anchors of (0.5 inch) white tape, one above and one below the injured joint.

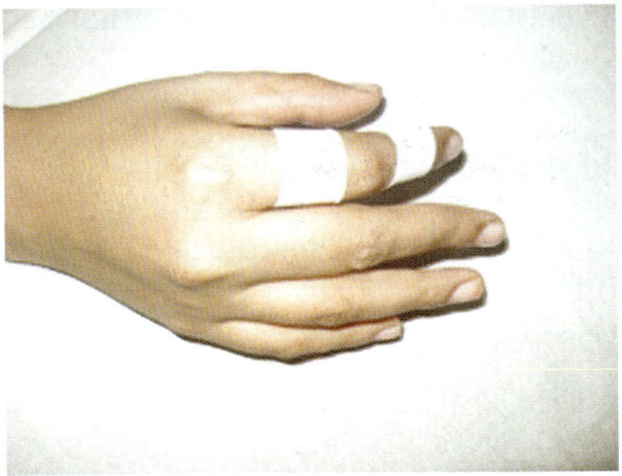

Fig. 11.9(c)

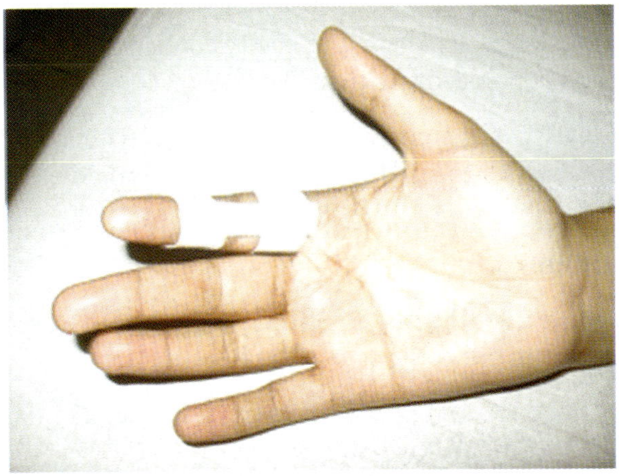

Fig. 11.9(d)

4. Apply a vertical strip of (0.5 inch) white tape from the distal anchor to the proximal anchor on the center of the vular (under) aspect of the finger, with strong tension; keeping the finger flexed about 20 degree.

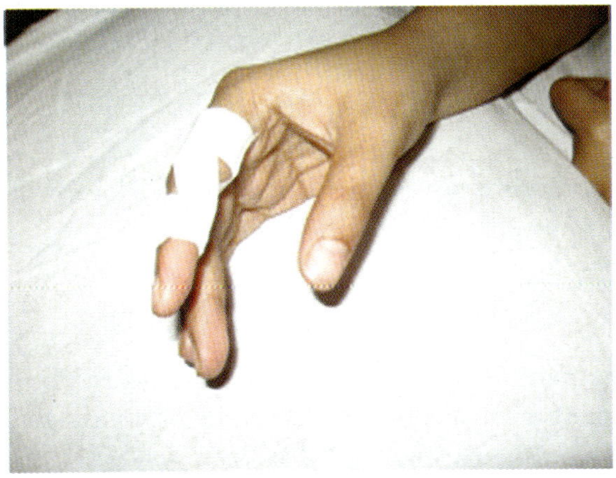

Fig. 11.9(e)

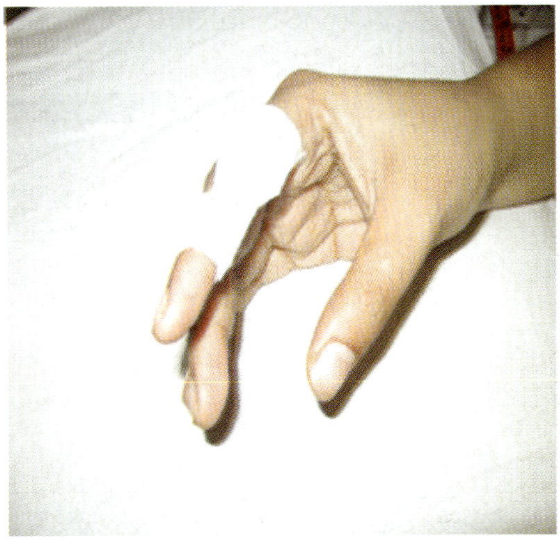

Fig. 11.9(f)

5. Apply a lateral X with two strips from the distal anchor to the proximal, with strong tension, forming the X on the lateral joint line.

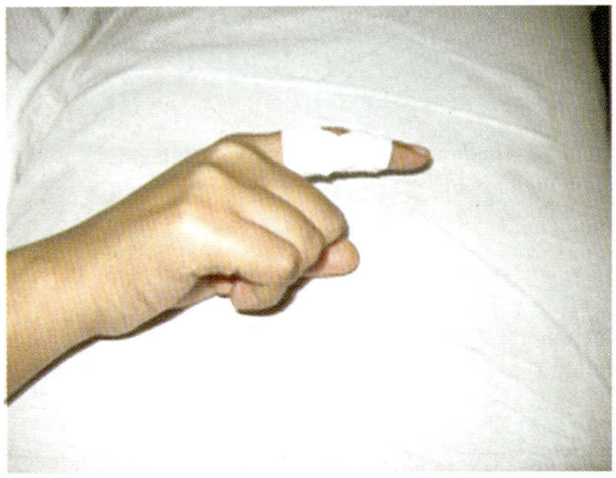

Fig. 11.9(g)

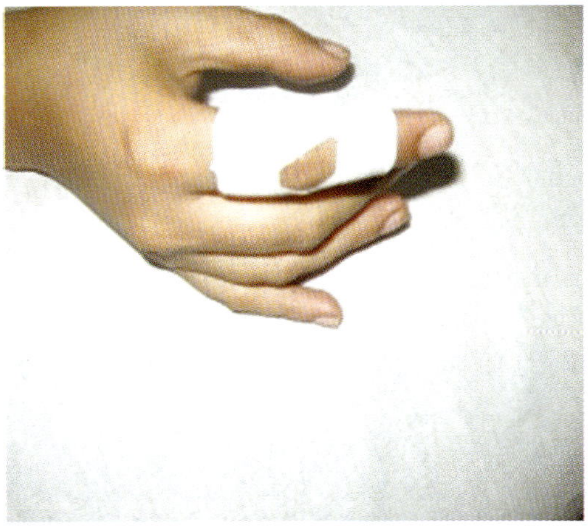

Fig. 11.9(h)

6. Repeat the above on the medial aspect, with the X lying on the medial joint line.

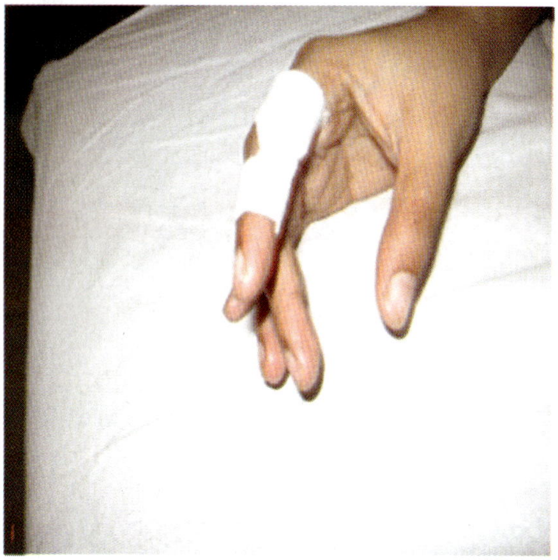

Fig. 11.9(i)

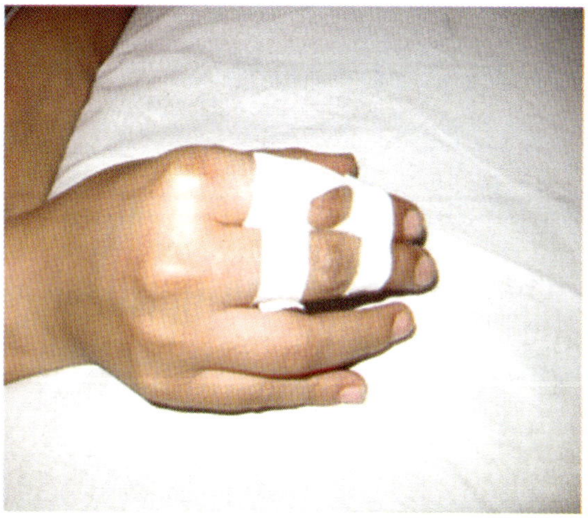

Fig. 11.9(j)

7. Repeat the anchors cover the ends of the vertical strips.
8. Perform a simple **"buddy taping"** technique by taping the injured finger to its neighbour.

NOTE: This step is useful for sports not needing full hand function (as in soccer), when the finger can function as a unit.

9. **Alternative method:** Apply a webbed **buddy taping** by keeping the injured digit slightly abducted (spread apart) while taping to its neighbour.

NOTE: This technique is useful for sports requiring full functional dexterity and use of individual fingers (as in basketball or volleyball). Note that more space is left between the fingers with this option.

GLOSSARY

Anchor: Anything which makes stable or secure, anything which is depended upon for support or security.

Basket weave: An interlocking of two or more strands resembling a basket.

Bursa: A pouch or sack like cavity containing synovial, located at points of friction.

Butterfly: A combination of taping strips with a typical form of wider top and bottom and narrow middle.

Buttress: A prop or support used to strengthen a structure.

Capsule: A fibrous container that envelops some structure of the body, as in a joint.

Cartilage: A tough, elastic form of connective tissue found on articulating bony spaces.

Caudal: Of, or pertaining to the tail or posterior part of the body, opposed to cranial.

Cranial: Of, or pertaining to the skull or superior part of the body, opposed to caudal.

Distal: Relatively remote from the center of the body or point of attachment, opposed to proximal.

Figure-8: A manoeuver that consist in tracing the Figure 8.

Horizontal strip: A strip which is placed level with the horizon, opposed to vertical strip.

Horseshoe: Padding made to resemble the U shape of a horseshoe.

Ligament: A band of firm fibrous connective tissue forming a connection between bones offering stability.

Lock: Any part that fastens, secures or holds something firmly in place.

Proximal: Relatively near the central position of the body, opposed to distal.

Stirrup: Any U shaped loop or piece.

Vertical strip: A strip that is placed perpendicular to the line of the horizon, opposed to horizontal strip.

REFERENCES

1. American Medical Association, *Standard nomenclature of athletic injuries A.M.A.,*Chicago,USA., 1966.
2. Austin, Karin, A., B.Sc. P.T, *Taping booklet. Physiotherapy International,* Montreal Canada, 1977.
3. Avis, Walter S., Editor, *Funk and Wagnall's standard college dictionary.* Fitzhenry and Whiteside Ltd., Toronto, Canada, 1978.
4. Backhouse, Kenneth M., O.B.E., V.R.D., and Hutchings R.T., *A Colour Atlas of Surface Anatomy.* Wolf Medical Publications, London, UK, 1986.
5. Bouchard Fernand, B.S.C. *Guide du soigneur.* Projet Perspective Jeunesse, Montreal, Canada, 1972.
6. British Columbia Sports Medical Council ,*British Columbia sports aid program, Victoria, B.C. Canada,1984.*
7. Cerney J.V.M.D. *Complete book of athlete taping techniques, Parker, New York, USA, 1972.*
8. Cyriax James, *Textbook of orthopeadic medical diagnosis of soft tissue injuries.*
9. Dixnon, Dwayne "spike" A.T., *The Dixonary of athlete training,* Bloomcraft-central printing Inc., Bloomington, Indiana, USA, 1965.
10. Griffith H. Winter M.D., The complete book of sports medicine, Warner Books Inc., New York, USA, 1979.
11. Griffith H.Winter, M.D., Complete guide to sports injuries. The body press, HP Books inc.,Tucson, Arizona, USA, 1986.
12. Head William F., M.S.F., Treatment of Atheletic injuries. Frank W. Horner Ltd.; Montreal, Canada, 1996.
13. Hess, Heinrich, Prof., Sportverletzungen. Luitpoldwerk, Munich, Germany, 1984.
14. Kapandgi I.A., The Physiology of the joints vol 1 & 2, Churchill Livingstone Edingburgh, Scotland, 1970.
15. Logan Gene A. Ph.D. R.P.T. and Logan Roland F., Techniques of Athletic Training. Franklin-Adams Press, Pasadena, California, USA, 1959.
16. Magee David J. Orthopaedic Physical Assessment, Saunders, Philadelphia, USA, 1987.
17. McConnell J., B.App. Sc. (phtg)., Grad. Dip., The Management of Chondromalacia Patallae: A long term solution, Physiotherapy, 32,(4), 1986, 215-223.
18. McMinn R.M.H. and Hutchings R.T., A Colour Atlas of Human Anatomy, Wolfe Publications, London, UK, 1977.
19. McMinn R.M.H., Hutchings R.T and Logan B.M. A Colour Atlas of Foot and Ankle Anatomy, Wolfe Medical Publications, London, UK, 1982.
20. Montag Hans-Jurgen and Asmussen Peter D., Functional Bandaging: A manual of bandaging technique. Beiersdorf Bibliothek, Hamburg, Germany, 1981.
21. Reid David C., Sports injury Assessment and Rehabilitation, Churchill Livingstone, New York, USA, 1992.
22. Williams Warwick (ed.) Gray's Anatomy. Churchill Livingstone Edinburgh, Scotland, 1970s.